# THE TORTURE DOCTORS

# THE
# TORTURE
# DOCTORS

## HUMAN RIGHTS CRIMES & THE ROAD TO JUSTICE

## STEVEN H. MILES, MD

Georgetown University Press / Washington, DC

179.7

The publisher is not responsible for third-party websites or their content. URL links were active at time of publication.

Library of Congress Cataloging-in-Publication Data
Names: Miles, Steven H., author.
Title: The Torture Doctors : Human Rights Crimes and the Road to Justice / Steven H. Miles, MD.
Description: Washington, DC : Georgetown University Press, 2020. | Includes bibliographical references and index.
Identifiers: LCCN 2019018296 (print) | ISBN 9781626167520 (hardcover : alk. paper) | ISBN 9781626167544 (ebook : alk. paper)
Subjects: LCSH: Torture—Moral and ethical aspects. | Physicians—Professional ethics. | Political prisoners—Medical care—Moral and ethical aspects. | Human rights.
Classification: LCC RA1122.8 .M55 2020 (print) | LCC RA1122.8 (ebook) | DDC 179.7—dc23
LC record available at https://lccn.loc.gov/2019018296
LC ebook record available at https://lccn.loc.gov/2019980385

⊗ This book is printed on acid-free paper meeting the requirements of the American National Standard for Permanence in Paper for Printed Library Materials.

21  20      9 8 7 6 5 4 3 2  First printing

Printed in the United States of America.

Cover design by Jeff Miller, Faceout Studio.
Cover images by Shutterstock and by Danil Novsky, Stocksy.

*I will go for the benefit of the ill,*

*while being far from all voluntary and destructive injustice.*

—Oath of Hippocrates, 450 BC

# CONTENTS

# Contents

# PREFACE

This book excavates a widespread, yet barely explored, medical specialty: the torture doctor. This is a work of medical anthropology. It describes how physicians collaborate with governments to create, inflict, and conceal practices that are intended to inflict severe pain and suffering. It recounts how human rights activists have pushed reluctant governments and medical associations to bring torture doctors to imperfect and rarely imposed forms of justice.

I am a recently retired professor of internal medicine. I practiced medicine and taught medical ethics for thirty-five years. The American Society of Bioethics and Humanities gave me its Lifetime Achievement Award. Work with refugees took me to places ripped apart by war and torture. I have met many torture survivors. They are even among the professors and students of my teaching hospital in Minnesota. They work in grocery stores, as journalists, or as taxi drivers. The US Office of Refugee Resettlement estimates that 500,000 torture survivors live in the United States, a total roughly equal to the number of persons with Parkinson's disease. Think about that number; every adult knows someone with Parkinson's disease. Stigma makes torture survivors invisible. Many are ashamed to tell their histories. Many people, even doctors, do not inquire about the cause of a person's nightmares or scars. Silence pushes torture below its rightful place on the national agenda, inhibiting survivors' rehabilitation and delaying reform of governmental and medical community policies.

People often ask those of us who rehabilitate survivors or who study torture, Why on earth would you do that? The question usually means that the topic is too distasteful or painful to contemplate. Ironically, many people who ask this question relax at home by watching torture for entertainment on a crime procedural or spy drama. For six years I served on the Board of the Center for Victims of Torture in Minneapolis. The center staff are as skilled as they are gracious and profound. I do not know of any who consume torture for entertainment.

In May 2004 I saw photographs of US soldiers abusing prisoners in Iraq. Questions came to mind: Where were the doctors of Abu Ghraib prison? Why had they not intervened when they saw the injuries? I sought the answer by reading tens of thousands of government pages that had been declassified by the American

Civil Liberties Union's relentless barrage of Freedom of Information Act requests. I expected to learn how the United States had suppressed doctors' protests. The truth was much more disheartening. Physicians and psychologists did not protest; rather, they assumed central roles in abusive interrogations. They designed and monitored torture. Pathologists falsified death certificates to prevent public discovery of torture. I wrote many articles and finally a book, *Oath Betrayed: America's Torture Doctors.* I indexed the declassified documents and posted them on a website at the University of Minnesota's Human Rights Library, where they were heavily used by lawyers and scholars.[1]

My interests then went global. I tracked the practices of torture doctors and the efforts to punish them around the world. I set up a website, The Doctors Who Torture Accountability Project. I am deeply grateful to Jay Lieberman, Mike Engelstad, and Laurie Walker, who designed the website. In 2015 I wrote an ebook, *Doctors Who Torture: The Pursuit of Justice,* which drew from some of the material on the website as I continued to compile information. The website was decommissioned at the end of 2017. Its files and many more are transferred to this book. My global study conformed with my experience in the United States; torture doctors rarely face accountability.

This book builds on two pathbreaking books that are now decades old. The American Association for the Advancement of Science published *The Breaking of Bodies and Minds: Torture, Psychiatric Abuse, and the Health Professions* in 1985.[2] The British Medical Association published *Medicine Betrayed: The Participation of Doctors in Human Rights Abuses* in 1992.[3] These books built on the anecdotes of their time and pointed to the need for study and reform.

Writing a book inevitably becomes an obsession. I am indebted to my wife, Joline Gitis, who is the special kind of person who can live with someone who pursues this kind of topic. Our gardens and dogs and horses (and I suppose cats) keep our home in equilibrium. Don Jacobs, my editor at Georgetown University Press, was encouraging and helpful. Sarah Deamer labored on the citations. The editors, production staff, and copyeditors at Georgetown University Press were supportive and skilled. I am grateful to the staff of Minneapolis's Center for Victims of Torture and of the Human Rights Program at the University of Minnesota Law School. I am deeply grateful for the support of the faculty and staff of the University of Minnesota's Center for Bioethics, who understood that this work is integral to the field of medical ethics. Each of these institutions embodies the humanity and intellectual energy of civil society. That spirit is the target of torture. That spirit alone will vanquish it.

# INTRODUCTION

Faustino Blanco Cabrera did not set out to be a torture doctor, but when his government turned to torture, that is what he became.

In 1976 Lieutenant Dr. Cabrera worked in the prisons of Argentina's military junta during its Dirty War. His job was to assess prisoners undergoing torture and tell the guards when to ease up on those who were supposed to live. He provided minor medical care to prisoners under torture who were supposed to live for a bit longer. He created and signed death certificates falsely asserting that imprisoned men or women who had been murdered by the state had died of natural causes. In 1983 the military junta fell from power and Cabrera slipped into private practice as a psychiatrist.

Twenty-three years later, in 2006, Cabrera's work as a torture doctor was discovered. He was tried and sent to prison. He was soon mysteriously freed and abandoned his family to move to another part of Argentina, where he practiced for six more years.[1] In 2013 his background was again discovered during a medical license renewal. The horrified medical staff revoked his hospital privileges on the grounds that he had misrepresented his past.[2] The provincial government accepted a petition declaring him persona non grata for "notorious moral unworthiness." As the petition put it, "his bad faith is shown by the fact that he has a medical license, hiding within the very healthcare system the abuse of which justifies this petition to expel him."[3]

An Argentine court tried Cabrera for torture, falsification of death certificates, and crimes against humanity. At the time his second trial began, one of Cabrera's psychiatry patients was a man with posttraumatic stress disorder (PTSD) from being tortured by the same junta that had employed Cabrera. The man's daughter was also one of Cabrera's patients. Her mental illness had resulted from the terror of living in hiding during her father's imprisonment. Until Cabrera's arrest, neither father nor daughter knew that their own physician had worked for the torturing regime that had traumatized them. In 2013 the daughter sat quietly in court watching her psychiatrist being sentenced to seven years in prison for being an accomplice to the terror that caused such suffering to her and her father.[4]

I learned of this story from an Argentine friend. A week after Cabrera had been sentenced, I began to compile materials for a book describing the practices of torture doctors and the efforts to bring them to justice.

Many people know that some Nazi doctors were tried after World War II for atrocities and vicious "experiments" on persons held in concentration camps. A few physicians were executed; a few were imprisoned; a few were acquitted. The vast majority of the Nazi doctors who were apprentices to the Holocaust were never brought before the bar of justice. Some people think that the trial of Nazi doctors at Nuremberg was the precedent for punishing Dr. Cabrera. The truth is not that straightforward. For thirty years after World War II, doctors had complete impunity as they collaborated with torture regimes around the world. In the mid-1970s an invigorated human rights movement began bringing government officials who violated human rights to justice in domestic tribunals in the countries where they had committed their crimes. It was the expanding reach of that development, and not the Nuremberg precedent, that snared Dr. Cabrera.

It is appalling but accurate to assert that many more physicians oversee torture than work to rehabilitate torture survivors. Torture doctors work for democracies such as the United States, Spain, and the United Kingdom. They assist sadistic practices in states like North Korea or Saudi Arabia. They devise techniques to minimize scars that might someday serve as evidence. They falsify medical records and death certificates to camouflage torture as the cause of an injury or of death.

This book tells how human rights advocates are trying to drive the threatening wedge of accountability between physicians and torturing regimes. This effort seeks to mobilize at least a few more physicians to refrain from lending their knowledge, skills, and medical privileges to the work of torture. Human rights advocates hope that some government official might pause in the midst of the ferocity and wonder, Will doctors betray our dirty work, if not out of a sense of justice, perhaps out of fear that their medical community or a court might call them to account for complicity?

This book describes an unexplored wreck. I have excavated only shards of the immense ruin of torture doctoring. Hundreds of anecdotes are described in these pages. But many more are missing. Documents have been destroyed or are hidden in sealed government archives. Witnesses, victims, and perpetrators have silently died. I have tried to avoid being gratuitously graphic. There are no photographs. The first half of this book is necessarily explicit, as it tells of the work and reasoning of torture doctors. Some readers might experience secondary trauma, especially if descriptions awaken memories of earlier assaults. Read in sips. The book lifts as it proceeds.

This collection of story fragments is not amenable to statistical analysis, solid causal inferences, or extrapolations. Yet a reader may fairly expect me to venture some opinions and working hypotheses for future scholars to explore. In meeting that expectation, I will be cautious to point out my limits, and I expect to live with future judgments on my efforts. The book compiles examples of what courts and medical licensing boards and medical associations have done to hold torture doctors accountable. I will build from that material to focus on what the medical profession can do to more effectively address the problem of the impunity of physicians who abet torture. I am not qualified to write a treatise on how domestic or international law might remedy this problem. My aim is to better equip civil society and the medical community to mobilize against torture doctors and thereby advance the cause of preventing torture.

This book's four parts unfold from describing the problem to describing the emerging solutions and finally to proposing further reforms.

Part 1, "Meet the Torture Doctors," summarizes what is known about doctors who torture. The first chapter, "Dr. Chand Sees a Burned Boy," tells the story of a doctor in Guyana whom the police summoned to see a boy they had brutally burned. Dr. Chand gave minimal treatment and left the boy in police custody without reporting the injuries. Chapter 2, "Who Are the Torture Doctors?" describes what is known about the attitudes and motivations of doctors who assist torture. The next chapter, "What Is Torture?" surveys the definitions of torture in a human rights context and summarizes research about the utility of torture for interrogation. Part 1's closing chapter, "What Is a Torture Doctor?" takes on the surprisingly complex task of defining a torture doctor.

Part 2, "A Time of Impunity," shows physician complicity with torture to be a global practice. Although few physicians abet torture, all torturing regimes rely on physicians to assist with or conceal torture. Chapter 5, "Judging the Nazi Doctors," recounts how the post–World War II Nuremberg vow to hold torture doctors accountable instantly gave way to the priorities of the Cold War. Chapter 6, "A Global Map of Torture Doctors," surveys worldwide practices of torture doctoring, including some regional or cultural variants. Chapter 7, "The Paradox of the United Kingdom," shows how the leading nation against physician complicity with torture has given impunity to its own torture doctors and how it disseminated the practice of medical monitoring of flogging throughout its former colonies, protectorates, and the Commonwealth.

Part 3, "Humanists and Healers," describes how an insurgent human rights movement took on the impunity of torture doctors. Chapter 8, "Humanists for Human Rights," sketches how nonphysicians articulated the right to be free of torture and, through fiction, introduced the reality of torture doctors to the public. Chapter 9, "Healers for Human Rights," is the story of how the antitorture human rights movement collaborated with clinical experts to create science-based forensic methods to bring torturers to justice. The final chapter of this section, "Organized Medicine's Condemn and Abide," surveys decades of post–World War II medical ethics codes that condemned physician complicity with torture, all the while carefully evading the task of how to hold torture doctors accountable.

Part 4, "The Dawn of Accountability," looks at the post–World War II record of instances where medical associations, licensing boards, or courts have undertaken to hold doctors accountable for complicity with torture. Chapter 11, "Innovations," looks at the initial wave of challenges to medicalized torture in the former Soviet Union and South Africa and then at a modest but remarkable cluster of cases in which torture doctors were held accountable as military juntas in Uruguay, Chile, Argentina, and Brazil collapsed. Chapter 12, "Globalization," traces the spread of accountability to encompass greater numbers of nations and physicians. It shows that despite the headlines, few torture doctors are ever called to account. A separate chapter is spent on "Impunity and the US War on Terror." In the United States medically supervised torture and complete impunity went hand in hand. The last chapter of this book, "Promoting Accountability," proposes how to evaluate progress in holding torture doctors accountable and how to better foster this process. Perhaps most important, it discusses why it is important to do so.

We can be firm in calling torture "evil" even as we recognize that torture doctors are largely banal careerists. Physicians' insights, motivations, and courage vary. Although it is not true that every physician can become a torturer, it is true that any regime can find the few doctors it requires to serve in its torture prisons. The integrity of the many physicians who will not serve in those prisons illuminates the baselessness of the excuses "I was afraid" or "I was under orders" that torture doctors offer after their regime has fallen and they are facing justice in public squares. Many torture doctors, such as those of the United States or Spain, have no legitimate fear of being tortured at all. Even in the most fascist regimes, there are always doctors who take enormous risks to expose torture and heal the survivors. Their brave and clinically expert witness illuminates maliciousness that was supposed to be beyond prosecution. Were it not for their professionalism, this book would not have been possible.

# PART I

## MEET THE TORTURE DOCTORS

# 1

# DR. CHAND SEES
# A BURNED BOY

On October 29, 2009, at 5:30 p.m., police summoned Dr. Mahendra Chand to attend to an injured prisoner. The police had detained a fourteen-year-old boy, Twyon Thomas, and brought him to the La Grange Police Station in Guyana on the north coast of South America. The police then transferred Twyon to the Leonora Police Station. They tied him to a chair, put a sack over his head, and secured it with a string around his neck. They beat him on his head and body in an effort to get him to confess to a homicide. There was no reason to believe Twyon was connected to a homicide, and no such charges were ever brought. Twyon felt a cold liquid running between his legs and onto his genitals. A police officer set the alcohol on fire, badly burning the boy.[1] The police then took Twyon to Vreed-en-Hoop Police Station and sent for Dr. Chand, who had been contracted to serve as a police doctor for the previous twelve years.

Dr. Chand arrived at the station and saw two policemen standing near his "patient," a boy with a bag over his head and wearing a shirt but with his burned genitals exposed for the physician to examine. Dr. Chand did not speak to the boy. He did not introduce himself. He did not ask the boy's name. He did not remove the bag over the boy's head. He focused on the burns as the police instructed. Dr. Chand saw what he later described as "first degree burns on the genital area, upper thighs and lower buttocks."[2] Newspaper photographs of the burned child show extensive second- and possibly third-degree burns through the skin and baring the muscle.[3] The doctor did not ask the police or his patient what had caused the burns. He did not look for other signs of torture, such as bruises from beatings under the boy's clothes or beneath the bag that concealed his face, even though the circumstances gave ample reason to believe that other injuries were present. He told police to treat the boy with oral antibiotics, analgesics, and an antiseptic cream. He did not make a medical note for the police or for his own office records.

He later claimed that he told the police to take the child to a hospital, but he did not record this instruction. The police denied that he made such a directive.[4] He did not report the abuse.[5] With no record of medical treatment, if the police had decided to disappear Twyon, the doctor would never have been connected to his death. Although the boy begged the police to take him to a doctor, the police detained him for four more days.

Finally, the police released the boy to his parents, who took him to a hospital for treatment. The Guyana Human Rights Association (GHRA) heard about the case, saw photographs of the burns, and learned of Dr. Chand's involvement. The organization protested to the Guyana Medical Council. The *Catholic Standard*, a diocesan newspaper, published the GHRA's point of view.[6] In response, the furious Dr. Chand wrote to the local newspaper stating that the GHRA "mischievously resorted to capricious, spurious and slanderous allegations which I suspect were crafted to satisfy some sordid or malicious intent." The rest of this letter deserves an unedited quotation:

> On the said day, I was called out by the police administration to see a patient about ten kilometers away from my home at six PM, a time very much outside my normal working hours. I readily agreed to go and see the patient. I would like to ask the GHRA whether acting beyond the call of duty is an act of callous indifference.
>
> On arrival at the Vreed-en-Hoop Police Station, I saw two ranks [police officers] in the inquiry area and introduced myself to them. After a short wait, I was presented with the said patient who was naked except for his head, which was covered with a bag. At this point, I must point out to the GHRA that the bag "was not tightened at the neck with a string" and that the patient was breathing comfortably.
>
> The injured area was exposed and that was solely my concern and focus. On examining the area I concluded that the patient was suffering from 1st degree [superficial] burns of the genital area, upper thighs and lower buttocks (5–9%). I did not see any other "areas of brutality" as alleged by the GHRA, nor did I see any signs of dehydration as alleged by the GHRA. I did mention verbally that the patient should have been carried to the hospital. Again I ask the GHRA whether this is callous indifference.
>
> I had a stamped prescription which I had walked with in anticipation of any medication that needed to be prescribed and I did prescribe antibiotics/ analgesics and an antiseptic cream. This fact was misleadingly left out of the article based on a release from the GHRA. Again, I ask whether this is callous indifference or complicity to torture.
>
> I never said that the patient was okay. In the given circumstances where no stationery was available and in a non-clinical setting, I did the best I could and acted with a clear conscience. I should like to make it clear that I have been practicing medicine in the Guyana Police Force for the past twelve years and I have always treated patients presented to me with care, sensitivity

and concern, whether they be ranks from the Guyana Police Force, detainees from the lock-ups or prisoners.

I have never ever knowingly or unknowingly encouraged torture, neither have I ever participated in any cover-up or "down-play." I left the Vreed-en-Hoop Police Station with the assumption that the patient would have been carried to the hospital as soon as it was possible to do so. To accuse me of a dereliction of duty and passive complicity with torture I consider to be most insulting and incorrect, and a sinister attempt to vilify and malign.

I refute the news article in the strongest possible terms and request that the GHRA stop forthwith associating me with direct, indirect, passive or active torture. I am not that kind of person, nor am I that kind of doctor. I urge that all of the unfounded and derisive remarks about me be retracted, and also that I be issued with an unconditional apology. Finally, I would suggest to the GHRA to cease casting aspersions in the media and to focus their energies more on some real humanitarian work in the prisons and underprivileged areas of the country.

Yours faithfully,

Mahendra Chand[7]

As has happened in many other torture doctoring cases, grateful patients wrote public testimonials attesting to Dr. Chand's compassion and skill.[8] Attesting to the fear of reprisals by the police in such situations, anonymous newspaper letters argued for censuring Dr. Chand.[9]

The Guyana Medical Council conducted an investigation, confidentially conveyed the results to Dr. Chand, and gave him one week to reply.[10] When he did not respond, the council censured Chand and suspended his medical license for two months for passive, silent complicity in torture.[11] The minister of health unexpectedly intervened and asked the council to reconsider the suspension.[12] According to one article, quoted here with its original paraphrasing and capitalization, the minister explained,

> "What is going through my head is one, the doctor was not part of any torture . . . the doctor was placed in a position that he had two options . . . One to walk away, remember the doctor took a Hippocratic oath of doing no harm because he did ask them to take off the bag [but the police refused]," the minister said.
>
> The minister said one of the options the doctor had was to walk away and "in which case we would have all sacrificed him because we would have said he should have taken care of the boy because that is his job. 'Do no harm' that is his Hippocratic oath."
>
> The second option he had was to treat the patient, which he did and made a prescription and referred him, the minister said.
>
> "So if those were his only two options he was damned if he did or damned if he didn't," the minister concluded.

"What I want to know from whomever, the medical council, I have asked them questions, what is any other possible options he had because maybe there was another option but right now I am only seeing two options and any doctor you would have put in the position would have ended up in trouble," the minister said.

"Unless there is another option I can't really blame the doctor, but I am not making the judgment I want somebody to tell me what other option . . . I am really at a point I am not certain anymore, you know when I first read the case I was as appalled as anybody else. I remain appalled but I am not quite sure if the doctor had a choice," the minister said.[13]

The council then revoked the two-month license suspension and reverted to simply censuring Dr. Chand.[14] The minister of health offered "no objection" to the council's censure.[15] The minister noted that Dr. Chand was loaned to the police by the Georgetown Public Hospital and suggested that the council "might want to consider any other action it might deem necessary."[16] The GHRA and several political parties characterized the censure as a "slap on the wrist." They accused the minister of health of depriving the Guyana Medical Council of the ability to enforce professional standards.

Remarkably, the boy and his mother bravely sued for damages. Even more remarkably, they prevailed. A judge awarded the teenager 6.5 million Guyanese dollars (about US$3,000), one-fourth of what his attorney had asked. Two police officers were ordered to personally pay the family US$365, more than two months' wages each.[17] The judge identified Dr. Chand as "the Police Surgeon," and her ruling stated that he "compounded the violations by what I consider to be a lack of sensitivity and professionalism." Twyon, his mother, and his lawyer have all gone into hiding. Criminal charges were brought against the police officers, but because Twyon did not show up to testify, the criminal charges were dropped.[18] The minority political party called for an investigation of police torture; the ruling party rebuffed that initiative. The department later promoted the two involved police officers, and the ensuing uproar led the vice president for public security to discharge the officers.[19] Sadly, there is evidence of ongoing medical complicity with torture in Guyana.[20]

This is a commonplace story of physician complicity with torture. The physician declined to enter a therapeutic relationship with the patient. Instead, his examination, treatment, record keeping, and reporting were confined to police requests rather than his patient's needs. The physician minimized the injuries in his reporting and did not ask the police or his patient about the cause of the burns. He contemptuously responded to criticisms by a human rights group. Under pressure from the human rights groups, a medical licensing board took up the matter and imposed a minor punishment. The government intervened to protect the physician. Yet, because a new human rights movement—one that is this book's subject—was under way, Dr. Chand was at least called to account.

# 2

# WHO ARE THE TORTURE DOCTORS?

The idea of a "torture doctor" is so extraordinary, so obscene that it almost defies comprehension. When people learn that I study this topic, they often exclaim, "What did you say?" thinking that they have misheard. Incredulity must be broken in order to see and undo the partnership between torture and doctoring. Physicians must be firmly on the side of safeguarding prisoners' health and monitoring for this most injurious of human rights violations. To demystify torture doctors, we must shift from a shocked, How could they? to more probing questions. Who are these people? What motivates them? Does being physicians psychologically insulate them from the horror of their work?

Such questions have no simple answers. There are a few biographical and autobiographical comments about torture doctors, but they are not compiled in a manner amenable to qualitative or quantitative analysis. There is scant research. We may not confidently generalize from the backgrounds, recruitment strategies, or political climates of small sets of torture doctors of one era or one national experience to those of other countries or other times. The results of small, brief, contrived studies—such as psychologist Stanley Milgram's oft-cited experiment in which forty adults were invited to the presumably safe grounds of a prestigious university and set up to falsely believe that a university faculty member was authorizing them to administer painful shocks—cannot be glibly applied to the completely different environment of filthy prisons where physicians see captives being grievously injured and murdered over several years.[1]

A few physicians have presided over autocratic torturing regimes.[2] François "Papa Doc" Duvalier, president of Haiti from 1957 until he died in 1971, was responsible for killing thirty thousand people and torturing countless more. Dr. Hastings Kamazu Banda, a US-educated physician, killed and tortured thousands of people in Malawi from 1961 to 1994 before he was forced from office, tried,

7

and acquitted of crimes against humanity. Dr. Bashar Hafez al-Assad presides over the torturing regime in Syria. Kurbanguly Berdymukhamedov of Turkmenistan and Félix Houphouët-Boigny of Ivory Coast (a locally trained physician) round out the list.

Then there are physicians who oversaw torture from positions as senior political officials. Such doctors often seem to subscribe to extreme nationalism or autocratic political ideologies. Several physician-politicians oversaw atrocities in the Yugoslav wars of the 1990s. Dr. Milomir Stakić quit his practice to become a senior municipal leader in Prijedor; he was sentenced to life in prison for establishing concentration camps, overseeing torture, and directing mass murder.[3] As president of the Bosnian-Serb Republic, Dr. Radovan Karadžić, a psychiatrist, assumed command of the Bosnian army and was eventually convicted of genocide and other crimes against humanity.[4] Dr. Milan Kovačević, a Serb anesthesiologist, died while being tried for genocide committed during his municipal administration.[5] Dr. Blagoje Simić, an internist, went into city politics and was later convicted and imprisoned for committing torture, setting up concentration camps, and committing other crimes against humanity.[6] One might speculate that senior political officials can easily distance themselves from the crimes committed by those under their orders. Simić protested his trial by saying that "he never hit anyone, never hurt anyone, and never pushed anyone. He said that he was leading and protecting his country."[7] The fact that none of these doctors were working as clinicians when they oversaw torture may account for why the texts of the verdicts focus on the crimes against humanity rather than on breaches of medical ethics.

In sentencing three doctors for war crimes committed during the 1994 Rwandan genocide, different courts mentioned medical ethics roughly in proportion to the proximity of the crimes to medical work. As the Rwandan genocide started, Dr. Gérard Ntakirutimana invited Tutsis, including some of his close friends, to take shelter at a hospital he managed. He stockpiled weapons for their slaughter, betrayed their location, and personally murdered people. In sending him to prison for murder and genocide, the court stated, "A doctor, he was one of the few individuals in his area of origin to have achieved a higher education and one of the rare schooled in Western universities. It is particularly egregious that, as a medical doctor, he took lives instead of saving them. He was accordingly found to have abused the trust placed in him in committing the crimes of which he was found guilty."[8] Dr. Clément Kayishema, a practicing surgeon, was a Rwandan governor who organized mass killings in nonclinical settings. In sentencing him to life in prison, the court called him "an educated medical doctor who betrayed the ethical duty that he owed to his community."[9] Dr. Eliézer Niyitegeka was not practicing medicine when, as Rwanda's minister of information, he helped organize the genocide. His life sentence makes no mention of medical ethics.[10] I am not so much interested in politicians who oversee torture, regardless of whether they have medical degrees.

I am much more interested in my medical colleagues who abet torture in the course of their clinical work. The vast majority of torture doctors are practicing clinicians. They neither hold nor aspire to political office. Some have military or police rank. Some are contracted to governments for part-time prison duties. Some have both government and private practices. Many are private practitioners whose ordinary work is interrupted when a relative or police officer brings a corpse or a tortured person for treatment and demands that the signs of torture not be noted in the medical examination, autopsy, or death certificate. Most torture doctors have no special professional distinction. A few are leaders in their medical communities. Dr. Leão Cabernite, for example, was president of the Psychoanalytic Society of Rio de Janeiro in Brazil (see chapter 11).[11]

There are three frames of reference for considering why doctors torture. First, one can look at the personal beliefs or personalities of physicians who do this work. Second, one can consider how a regime socializes some physicians to submerge their professionalism to complicity with torture. Finally, one can consider external pressures (e.g., fear or orders) often invoked as excuses for abetting torture.

It is simplistic to assert that torture doctors are by their nature psychopathic sadists looking for the opportunity to torture. Physicians, like anyone else, are capable of affirming the most grandiose and destructive forms of patriotism. The Nazi ideology of "race hygiene" attracted doctors to carry out genocidal eugenics policies to improve the genetic health of the population. Under this system, the state cataloged and ranked the genetic health of individuals to promote births by genetically "superior" persons and to sterilize or eliminate the others. Physicians responded to the power and prestige of this pseudoscience by joining the Nazi Party early and in great numbers.[12] Adolf Hitler's mythic "Thousand Year Reich," like Slobodon Milošević's "Greater Serbia," claimed to confer a heroic authority that transcended ordinary ethical norms. It is not surprising to hear a Nazi doctor, inflated by the mythic gas of the Thousand Year Reich, say, "The moment an individual is absorbed into the concept of a collective body, every demand which is put to that individual has to be absorbed into the concept of a collective system. Therefore, the demands of society are placed above every human being as an entity and this entity, the human being, is completely used in the interests of that society."[13] It is impossible to understand how Dr. Amílcar Lobo Moreira da Silva did not realize that he was merely a cog in the grubby Brazilian prison in which he oversaw the brutal torture of hundreds of prisoners in the 1970s. And yet he wrote, "Man has used torture and assassination for thousands of years and permitted it as long as it is socially organized. It is but an instant between the Inquisition's torture and murder of the Jews and the Nazi regime's similar actions forty years ago. This is human nature; I am not ashamed to be part of it."[14]

Many torture doctors act as if they believe they are serving necessary national policies.[15] Psychological research finds that a proclivity for right-wing aggression is associated with a constellation of high fear of the dangers of the world, tough-mindedness, prejudice against outgroups, and willingness to conform to a hierarchy of dominance (in which outgroups are stigmatized as being at the bottom).[16] A Chilean doctor, himself imprisoned, heard prison doctors justify the abuses and quoted a young prison doctor speaking "to me in a rather aggressive manner: 'What do you expect? We are at war,' taking for granted obviously that the practice of torture should be acceptable in case of war."[17] A patriotic doctor blinded by such nationalism can even rationalize dissecting people alive as being necessary to his country's war interests.[18] Such patriotism basks in the reflected light of proximity to power. Lobo's wife said, "I was dazzled when General Sylvio Frota [minister of the Brazilian army] appeared in the office. . . . I thought it was fantastic that Amilcar was receiving the attention of someone so important."[19]

Many torture doctors ferociously reject the relevance of medical ethics and human rights to their work. This rejection means that human rights is simply a political criticism and that medical ethics codes against torture have no substance. Nazi doctor Karl Brandt stood on the gallows and shouted that the Nuremberg conviction was "nothing but political revenge. . . . It is no shame to stand on this scaffold. I served my Fatherland." Nazi doctors Karl Gebhardt (former head of the German Red Cross), Joachim Mrugowsky, and Aribert Heim had similarly combative last words.[20] Professor Andrei Snezhevsky, who directed the Soviet psychiatric system that abused dissidents, complained to the head of England's Royal College of Physicians, "The Royal College has taken a very dubious function of intervening into the inner affairs of national psychiatric associations and using mentally ill patients for political purposes."[21] He called the censure by the World Medical Association (WMA) of Soviet psychiatry for abusing dissidents a "malicious concoction."[22] The Serb doctors cited previously expressed contempt for being tried for crimes against humanity. The American Psychological Association's Presidential Task Force on Psychological Ethics and National Security specifically refused to consider medical ethics or human rights as relevant to its work in support of psychologists who oversaw brutal interrogations (see chapter 13). Dr. Larry James, a US military psychologist who played several roles in creating and then reforming the war on terror program for abusive interrogations, expressed his disdain for the Red Cross prison inspections:

> The International Committee of the Red Cross (ICRC) consistently takes a critical view of the United States. Like most other soldiers, I saw the ICRC representatives as a bunch of radical left do-gooders, mostly from Europe, who were as interested in giving America a black eye as they were in truly helping the innocent. Every ICRC rep I met had long, disheveled '60s and '70s hairstyles as well as Birkenstock sandals—the consummate hippie motif. They thought all of the detainees were completely innocent and only needed to be hugged more. I was seen as a devil by them, supposedly helping interrogators craft abusive interrogation practices. I hadn't been in Abu Ghraib long before the ICRC accused me of torturing prisoners. . . . It was the ICRC who concocted the story of medical torture.[23]

James Mitchell, a psychologist and one of the architects of the US Central Intelligence Agency (CIA) war on terror torture program, complained about media criticism: "It's like being caught up in a Kafka novel. . . . They're just interested in burning down the CIA and smearing the names and reputations of people who died protecting this country."[24] The Iraqi torture doctor Mohammed Kassim Al-Byati refused to attend his judgment by the British Medical Council, telling a reporter, "So, if you think that treating people who were tortured was a crime, it's up to you."[25] South Africa's Dr. Benjamin Tucker, who was suspended for three months for neglecting the fatally tortured Stephen Biko, wrote curtly to the medical council, "I have been advised that in order to be re-admitted I have to apologize. I hereby do so."[26]

Beyond an affinity for autocratic politics, many of these quotes express not only rage and contempt for human rights but also a feeling of being victimized by human rights and medical ethics criticisms. One hears this feeling of victimization in Chand's letter to the newspaper cited in chapter 1. A torture doctor's sense of being aggrieved can even extend to the prison in which he or she works. In Argentina Dr. Julio César Caserotto was on trial for torture (he died before the verdict). His midwife testified that he had said of a woman on whom he was performing postoperative care after a cesarean section in prison, "I do not know why we take care of them so much if we throw them into the river later on."[27]

The torture prison differs in every way from lovely Linsly-Chittenden Hall, where the Milgram experiment took place. Linsly-Chittenden Hall is in peaceful New Haven on the campus of the prestigious Yale University; it is most decidedly not in a culture of political terror where people inexplicably disappear and then sometimes return with physical scars and nightmares that mute their speech. An advertisement drew forty adult volunteers to Linsly-Chittenden Hall. They were told that they would be advancing the cause of science by participating in a study of the effects of electric shocks on learning. A "scientific authority" directed these volunteers to administer shocks to an actor who screamed increasingly loudly as the (imaginary) electric shocks supposedly increased in intensity.[28] Milgram concluded that the volunteer "torturers" surrendered their morality to authority. Unlike Milgram's volunteers, the consciences of real torturers are never assuaged with the belief that they are acting with the consent of a "victim" at an elite university in a democracy.[29]

Prisons where executions are performed offer some insights into the adaptive socialization of torturers. Executioners are most likely to endorse the moral and social necessity of executions, to dehumanize prisoners, and to deny personal responsibility for the deaths. The guards, ministers, and social workers working with death row prisoners are less extreme on all these measures. With time, the staff members who are more peripheral to the execution assume views more akin to those of the executioners.[30] Their sense of personal (or professional) responsibility molds itself to the institutional milieu. This response is similar to Erving Goffman's observations in other "total institutions," or organizations that socialize staff to institutional purposes and norms of behavior.[31] The culture of total institutions stigmatizes, segregates, disempowers, and dehumanizes prisoners. In a torture prison, disparities of power and loss of empathy for dehumanized victims lubricate the machine. There may be important differences between the torture apprenticeships of nonphysician soldiers and physicians. A small Greek study of how soldiers were trained to torture found that they were selected for patriotism, schooled by brutal initiations, and then introduced to torture by witnessing it, serving food to victims, participating in mass beatings, and then taking on managerial roles.[32] I do not know of any similar apprenticeship for physicians.

Dr. Robert Lifton, a psychiatrist who studied Nazi doctors and soldiers who committed atrocities during war, suggested that persons in "atrocity-producing situations" undergo "doubling," by which they create two selves: one for personal life and one for their work life.[33] In this way, a person is able to be a loving parent at home and a torturer while working at a prison. Lifton wrote that doubling is not a psychosis, a personality disorder, or a coerced adaptation. His view was based on Nazi doctors who turned the work of murder on a gargantuan scale into a technical problem to be solved to advance the Reich.[34] Peter Vesti and Niels Lavik similarly suggested that torture prisons put doctors at risk of abetting torture by having supportive senior colleagues groom medical staff and by dehumanizing prisoners in the service of a grand ideological justification for the torture.[35] A physician who worked with the infamous Auschwitz doctor Josef Mengele to solve the difficulties of industrial-scale murder referred to Mengele as a "commendable" optimistic man of "integrity" who "was merely acting consistently with the Auschwitz principles."[36] Philip Zimbardo, the psychologist who conducted the Stanford prison experiment in which students were divided into guards who became abusive and prisoners, said that abusive prison rules supply rationalizations to manage the moral dissonance between life inside and outside the prison.[37] If Zimbardo and Lifton are correct, one might expect to see torture doctors redefine what it means to be "medical professionals" so as to decrease the contradiction between their roles as healers and their collaboration with torture.

Some torture doctors imbue their work with a sham medical professionalism. Some rationalize their work as therapeutic. In chapter 1 Dr. Chand asserted that he acted therapeutically as he abandoned the young boy to the police who had beaten and burned him. Chilean torture survivor Jacobo Timerman describes his torture doctor, whom he later testified against:

> Two days have gone by without torture. The doctor came to see me and removed the blindfold from my eyes. I asked him if he wasn't worried about my seeing his face. He acts surprised.
>
> "I'm your friend. The one who takes care of you when they apply the machine. Have you had something to eat?"
>
> "I have trouble eating. I'm drinking water. They gave an apple."
>
> "You're doing the right thing. Eat lightly. After all, Gandhi survived on much less. If you need something call me."
>
> "My gums hurt. They applied the machine to my mouth."
>
> He examines my gums and advised me not to worry. I'm in perfect health. He tells me he is proud of the way I withstood it all.[38]

Al-Byati worked for the Iraqi Intelligence Agency at a prison where "horrific atrocities were committed." He knew his patients were tortured. When they were brought to him, "they looked like somebody who had a big accident." He gave minimal treatment and knew that the prisoners would be tortured again. As he put it, "For me, I was the one who was helping them." He stated with some pride that "they were alive when he left," and therefore he claimed that he had done his job "as a doctor."[39] Dr. Hans Eisele, a Nazi physician at Buchenwald concentration camp, was twice sentenced to death for lethal experiments and sadistic torture. In his autobiography, *Listen to the Other Side Too*, he claimed to be a humane Christian. Soviet physicians rationalized their treatment of dissidents with the diagnosis "sluggish schizophrenia," a nonexistent disease with the cardinal symptom of belief in social reform.[40] In Chile a torture doctor told Dr. Alfredo Jadresic, an imprisoned colleague, "that he had nothing to do with what was going on in the country, he was there to carry out his professional duties as a military doctor." Jadresic added, "several [doctors] showed their sympathy for the tortured prisoners and promised they would do something."[41]

A few torture doctors reduce the dissonance between their medical role and their complicity with the torture by rationalizing that they are advancing medical science. Japanese and German doctors during World War II saw themselves as patriotic physicians working in the service of science.[42] Japan and Germany studied biological warfare with prisoners. Nazis studied how long men could stay alive in ice water using various kind of protective gear for seamen. The list is endless. Dr. Gerhard Rose, who was sentenced to life in prison by the Nuremberg tribunal, asserted, "Works of that nature ["experiments" giving prisoners lethal infections with typhus and malaria] have nothing to do with politics or with ideology, but they serve the good of humanity. The same problems and necessities can be seen independently of any political ideology everywhere, where the same dangers of epidemics have to be combated."[43] Dr. Carl Peter Vaernet, a Danish physician who collaborated with the Nazis, implanted testosterone-secreting glands to "cure" gay prisoners at Buchenwald.[44] Dr. Karasawa Tomio, whom the Soviets sentenced for gruesome experiments on prisoners of the Japanese, stated, "I shall justify it as a doctor who engages in the benevolent art."[45]

Collegiality among torture doctors reinforces membership in a deviant medical community. In Argentina, physicians shared ideas, leading to the widespread practice of falsifying birth certificates of tortured and murdered women who delivered babies while imprisoned (see chapter 11). Darius Rejali proposes that because torture has no scientific foundation, collegiality among torturers becomes the means by which local practices are taught.[46] Brazilian psychiatrist Dr. Leão Cabernite oversaw torture as he psychoanalyzed his trainee-patient Dr. Amílcar Lobo, who followed in his mentor's footsteps to become a torture doctor.[47] Lobo went on to conduct horrific classes in torture for his colleagues. One female prisoner recalled,

On 20 October, two months after my imprisonment and already sharing the cell with other prisoners, I served as a guinea pig for a torture class. The teacher, in front of his students, did demonstrations with my body. It was a type of practical class, with some theoretical tips. I took electric shocks while hung in the "pau de arara" [hung upside down by a pole under the bent knees with the feet tied to the arms] and I heard the teacher say, "this is the most efficient technique." I think the teacher was right.

As I began to feel ill, the class was interrupted and I was taken to the cell. A few minutes later, several officers entered the cell and asked for the doctor to measure my blood pressure. The girls screamed, begged, trying in vain to prevent the class continuing. The doctor Amilcar Lobo's answer, in front of the torturers and all of us, was, "She can still take it." And, indeed, the class continued.[48]

Dr. Leo Alexander, the medical adviser in the Nazi doctors' trial, concluded that a morally lazy careerism lies at the core of most physicians who abet torture.[49] The doctors are rewarded with ranks and promotions, and even medical education.[50] I concur with Alexander's assessment. Rationalizing participation in torture by relying on one's title—i.e., therapist or researcher—and lazily accepting that this is how medicine is practiced in war exemplify sham medical careerism.

Finally, we must consider the claim that fear is the force majeure that coerces doctors to torture. When Dr. Solimaro was a prisoner at risk of torture in Chile, an army officer asked his medical opinion as to how to keep prisoners from dying of electric shock torture. The officer said we are "losing too many people." The terrified Solimaro told the officer that medicine had no such guarantees and that the torture should be stopped.[51] Solimaro also noted that doctors working for the torture prison "pretended to ignore what they saw and appeared very much guarded of talking about it."[52] The fear argument has most weight when a doctor is also a prisoner, as was the case for a few Jewish physicians held in Nazi death camps.[53] However, prisoners also collaborate with torture, as in the example of Anne Spoerry. Spoerry was a medical student when the Nazis arrested her soon after she joined the French Resistance. She was sent to Ravensbrück concentration camp, where she became an informer, torturer, and executioner, fitting the careerist model. After the war she finished her medical education. She was called to account and exiled from France for her collaboration with the Nazis. She went to Africa, where she became a doctor to the poor and remained quiet about her past.[54]

Threats are rarely used to coerce doctors. A senior Nazi official asked two physician experts in aviation medicine to perform experiments like those that resulted in other physicians' being punished at Nuremberg. Both refused on moral grounds to abuse human subjects and faced no retaliation.[55] Gerhard Küntscher, a Nazi orthopedic surgeon, perfected his enormous surgical advance for healing broken femurs by operating on injured soldiers of all sides. He refused to speed up his work by taking concentration camp prisoners, whose legs would have been broken for him.[56] Chilean doctors could decline to accept careers in torture prisons and work instead in the other parts of the health care sector.[57] Research indicates that fear of torture played no role in the complicity of physicians from the United Kingdom or Israel with torture.[58] Saddam Hussein asked some Iraqi doctors to torture people of their own ethnic group as a test of loyalty but not to get the doctor to pursue a career in torture.[59] I know of one case in which the Nazis led a physician to fear that his loyalty was being questioned; he proved himself with the "blood-cement" of exceptional viciousness.[60] Chapter 13 discusses how the clinicians who worked for the US war on terror interrogation centers could volunteer for "enhanced interrogation" services but had the option of asking to be reassigned.

Most regimes can ill afford to alienate their medical communities by coercing physicians to assist torture. Most torturing countries have shortages of physicians because physicians emigrate away from political terror and the poverty of autocratic regimes. Regimes know that a persecuted medical community can communicate and collaborate with global human rights organizations to compile and share evidence of torture. Furthermore, torturing regimes do not need many prison physicians. A couple hundred of Nazi Germany's 180,000 doctors worked in the concentration camps.[61]

In judgments that were contemporaneous with the events, the WMA (in evaluating Nazi doctors) and the Chilean Medical Association rejected fear as excusing medical complicity with torture.[62] The most compelling evidence against the excuse is the simple fact that a huge majority of doctors do not collaborate with torture. In fact, physician resistance to complicity with torture and the resulting collaboration with human rights organizations leaked many of the anecdotes in this book. When Dr. Muhammad Tahir in Pakistan was presented with the tortured body of a teenage boy and directed to prepare an autopsy report that did not record the torture, he told a newspaper, "I refused to compile a false post mortem report in order to save the culprits. I have taken an Oath to serve people not officials."[63]

In most cases the torturer's plaint "I was coerced" joins "I am being politically persecuted" and "If I did not do it, someone else would have done so" as self-excusing rationalizations. Claiming coercion is a way to deny personal responsibility. Brazil's Lobo, who tortured an estimated five hundred prisoners, was not coerced. His wife, the woman who bragged about how thrilled she was about his proximity to power, defended him this way: "Forgive him; my husband had no courage. . . . [He] attended the tortured, yes but was not responsible for the torture. Was he negligent? If so, it was because he did not ask anyone for help. I want someone to tell me who he could have turned to and where he could have sought asylum. He was punished as an accomplice. The entire blame belongs to the accomplice?"[64]

## A Coda on Dual Loyalty Ethics

Dual loyalty ethics posits that physician complicity with torture can to some degree be justified or at least understood because physicians are seeking a difficult balance between conflicting loyalties to the patient and to the government. Some dual loyalty dilemmas are reasonably well worked out. For example, the duty to respect a sick person's autonomous choices can be weighed against the threat of allowing a serious infection to spread to the broader public. In this case a doctor might get legal permission to isolate and treat an uncooperative patient with tuberculosis. The proceedings for obtaining permission must respect due process, and the doctor must implement the least restrictive isolation possible (e.g., the shortest isolation period) until the risk to the public is gone. Given that torture is illegal under international law, causes diverse harms, and has no demonstrated utility, dual loyalty ethics does not excuse physician complicity with torture.[65] Some might argue that a doctor in a torture prison may justifiably ease pain caused by torture or intervene to prevent death, for example, from lacerations caused by torture. However, since these treatments enable the torture to continue, they are not excused by dual loyalty ethics. Physicians instead must honestly record the nature, severity, and cause of injuries; endeavor to remove the tortured prisoner from the prison system; and report the abuses to human rights authorities. Ethics codes on this point are covered in chapter 10.

# 3

# WHAT IS TORTURE?

In common crime news a "torturer" is a sadistic person who confines and repeatedly attacks a victim. Torturers are criminals; they kidnap, assault, rape, and murder. The torturer and victims know that discovery will lead to arrest and prosecution. In human rights laws and in the related medical ethics codes, "torture" has a specialized definition.

Torture: any act by which severe pain or suffering, whether physical or mental, is intentionally inflicted on a person for such purposes as obtaining from him or a third person information or a confession, punishing him for an act he or a third person has committed or is suspected of having committed, or intimidating or coercing him or a third person, or for any reason based on discrimination of any kind, when such pain or suffering is inflicted by or at the instigation of or with the consent or acquiescence of a public official or other person acting in an official capacity. It does not include pain or suffering arising only from, inherent in or incidental to lawful sanctions.
—United Nations' Convention against Torture and Other Cruel,
Inhuman or Degrading Treatment or Punishment[1]

Torture: the deliberate, systematic or wanton infliction of physical or mental suffering by one or more persons acting alone or on the orders of any authority, to force another person to yield information, to make a confession, or for any other reason.
—WMA's Declaration of Tokyo[2]

Cruel, inhuman or degrading treatment or punishment: should be interpreted so as to extend the widest possible protection against abuses, whether physical or mental, including the holding of a detained or imprisoned person in conditions which deprive him, temporarily or permanently, of the use of

any of his natural senses, such as sight or hearing, or of his awareness of place
and the passing of time.

—United Nations' Body of Principles for the Protection of All
Persons under Any Form of Detention or Imprisonment

1. Torture means any act by which severe pain or suffering, whether physical
   or mental, is intentionally inflicted by or at the instigation of a public official on a person for such purposes as obtaining from him or a third person
   information or confession, punishing him for an act he has committed or
   is suspected of having committed, or intimidating him or other persons. It
   does not include pain or suffering arising only from, inherent in or incidental to, lawful sanctions to the extent consistent with the Standard Minimum
   Rules for the Treatment of Prisoners.
2. Torture constitutes an aggravated and deliberate form of cruel, inhuman or
   degrading treatment or punishment.

—United Nations' Principles of Medical Ethics Relevant to the Role
of Health Personnel, Particularly Physicians, in the Protection
of Prisoners and Detainees against Torture, and Other Cruel,
Inhuman or Degrading Treatment or Punishment[3]

As in crime news, torturers intentionally inflict severe physical or psychological
pain or suffering. However, torture as a human rights violation differs in that it
is authorized by a government with the aim to interrogate, punish, deter future
crime, or terrorize or suppress dissidents or minorities. Protected by government
policy, torturers have little fear of prosecution, and the victims' suffering is compounded by the loss of hope for rescue, justice, or compensation. Victims and their
loved ones know that the government will protect torturers from punishment, a
protection called "impunity" (see part 2). The Association for the Prevention of
Torture has extensive resources about the definition of torture.[4] Prisoners who
see doctors abetting torture are especially aggrieved. Nazi death camp survivor
Elie Wiesel put it this way: "Am I naive in believing that medicine is still a noble
profession, upholding the highest ethical principles? For the ill, doctors still stand
for life. And for us all, hope."[5]

One may distinguish extrajudicial torture, which is wantonly inflicted by
police or soldiers, from judicial torture, which is imposed as a judicial sentence.
Police or soldiers inflict extrajudicial torture regardless of whether a person has
been properly arrested, charged, convicted, or sentenced.[6] They may inflict it as
a form of social discrimination (e.g., sodomizing homosexuals with batons), as a
means to extract a confession, or as a form of vigilantism. The techniques of extrajudicial torture are limited only by the ingenuity, equipment, caseload, or fatigue of
the torturers. Judicial torture is imposed as a sentence after conviction for a crime.
It is specified from a small list of potential punishments. For example, a court
might sentence a thief to "twenty-five full force lashes on the back with a rattan

cane." Human rights groups report that all countries that allow judicial torture also tolerate extensive extrajudicial torture. Physicians are complicit with extrajudicial torture as described in the account of Dr. Chand (see chapter 1) and with judicial torture such as flogging (see chapter 6).

Governments rationalize torture as punishing criminals, upholding orthodoxies, deterring crime, obtaining information, or suppressing insurrections, minorities, or dissidents.[7] Malise Ruthven notes that torture often rests on a deeper social allegory.[8] He argues that leaders of torturing nations often raise the specter of the nation as being threatened by a "Grand Conspiracy." In this context torture is needed to battle a transcendentally powerful evil (Communists, counter-revolutionaries, Islamo-fascists, infidels, etc.), and to terrify and unify society for the struggle. For example, Hitler used anti-Semitism both to mobilize a political base and to justify genocide. The threat posed by the Grand Conspiracy justifies voiding ordinary laws or norms against torture. News media, education, and even entertainment (e.g., television shows like *24*) propagandize the necessity and efficacy of torture. Laws then define "the enemy" as a special criminal class without rights. Secret prisons where human rights, due process, ordinary penal codes, or international laws do not apply are designated.

Nations contrive artful policies to explain why their torture is not real torture. Some places assert that amputating a thief's hand is a holy mandate and therefore beyond the judgment of human laws. During the war on terror, the US government crafted novel legal interpretations to say that waterboarding (which it had previously defined as torture) was not torture, in part because death and organ failure were not intended (see chapter 13).[9] Partly to forestall such wordplay, laws and ethics codes against torture define a lesser level of abuse, often called "cruel, inhuman, or degrading treatment or punishment" (see the UN definition earlier in this chapter). The intricacies of the distinctions between "torture" and "cruel, inhuman, or degrading treatment or punishment" are discussed elsewhere.[10] These distinctions are not relevant to this discussion, because medical codes bar physicians from complicity with both of them. For example, the WMA's Declaration of Tokyo, cited earlier, states, "The physician shall not countenance, condone or participate in the practice of torture or other forms of cruel, inhuman or degrading procedures."

## Conditions of Confinement as Torture

Inhumane prison conditions test the distinction between "torture" and "cruel, inhuman, or degrading treatment or punishment." This issue is germane to prison health professionals because the UN Principles of Medical Ethics states that torture "does not include pain or suffering arising only from . . . lawful sanctions," outlined in the Standard Minimum Rules for the Treatment of Prisoners. So far, this book has depicted torture as an official inflicting pain on a prisoner. However, a physician might work in a prison milieu that is so severe as to itself constitute torture or cruel, inhuman, or degrading treatment or punishment. Human rights advocates are clarifying when conditions of confinement constitute abuse. The issues are illustrated by the roles of physicians treating prisoners in solitary confinement (see chapter 10) or working in some refugee detention centers.

Nations often design miserable refugee detention centers to deter refugees from coming to the nation or to convince them to abandon their requests for asylum or immigration. Refugees' rights are foundational for assessing the conditions of detention centers. International law affirms that people have the right to seek asylum in other countries, to have their basic needs met while pleas for asylum are evaluated, to have timely and fair review of petitions for asylum, and to not be involuntarily deported to places where there is reason to believe that their lives are in danger.[11] Those human rights define the complementary duties of nations that refugees enter.

To deter the approach and prevent the entry of refugees from Southeast Asia, the Australian government intercepts incoming refugee boats and inters the passengers in harsh centers on neighboring islands that are sovereign nations.[12] Even though the Australian government has custody of the boat people as it transfers them to the offshore centers, Australia does not grant the refugees the rights of asylum seekers on the argument that they did not reach Australian soil. The United Nations describes these detention centers as being so far from meeting basic human needs as to inflict torture or cruel, inhuman, or degrading treatment.[13] Physicians in the centers are underequipped for treating medical conditions, even those caused by the centers' harsh conditions.[14] Only a few severely ill refugees are transferred to Australian hospitals for care. On occasion physicians have refused to discharge unwell patients in order to prevent them from being transported back to the offshore prisons without being allowed to submit a claim for asylum.

Australia's medical community has collaborated with domestic and international human rights groups to denounce the policy.[15] Doctors for Refugees formed shortly after the first detention center opened in 2013.[16] Human rights groups often cite unnamed physicians as providing some of their information about conditions in the detention centers. In 2019 Dr. Nick Martin, who was fired because of his human rights advocacy, received an international award for his whistleblowing on the inhumane conditions in the Nauru detention center.[17] Australia and the host governments of the imprisoning islands have raided relief organizations serving refugees to prevent them from reporting abuses to human rights organizations.[18] In 2015, two years after the prisons opened, Australia passed the Border Force Bill, stating that anyone, including doctors, who reported conditions and human rights abuses in the detention centers could be imprisoned for disclosing state secrets.[19] In July 2016 physicians groups sued to overturn that bill. The government soon issued a revocable executive order exempting doctors and health professionals (but not other aid workers) from its provisions. Some Australian doctors argue for boycotting the offshore prisons, although Australia could alternatively hire replacement clinicians from neighboring developing countries who would be less inclined to protest human rights violations.[20]

In 2017 the United States precipitously began separating thousands of children from their refugee parents as part of a larger policy to deter asylum seekers.[21] The separations were irregularly and inconsistently documented, and the government substantially understated the number of children who were taken from relatives.[22] The separations, inhumane in their conception, were so chaotic that records associating children with parents were lost, destroyed, or never created in the first place.[23] Children and families were distraught. Some parents were deported without their children as young as three years old. Children were sexually abused or died in the isolated custodial centers. The United Nations High Commissioner for Human Rights opined, "Detention of children is punitive, severely hampers their development, and in some cases may amount to torture. . . . Children are being used as a deterrent to irregular migration, which is unacceptable."[24] Numerous federal and state rulings against the detention have not been effective.[25] In my view these separations are akin to a form of torture or cruel, inhuman, or degrading treatment in which family members are abused in front of each other.

US medical associations have condemned the policy of separating children from families and stressed the likelihood of grave harms such as PTSD.[26] However, those organizations have not reminded doctors of their personal accountability to law and standards of care regarding these children. For clinicians working in the detention centers, the challenges are more pressing than simply denouncing the policy. Physicians oversee drugging and restraining agitated, panicked children without the legally required oversight and approval of court-appointed guardians and judicial review.[27] They apparently sign Fitness to Transfer forms as children are sent to other centers (even in distant states) without confirming that a relative has been informed of the location of the child or knowing whether a relative is able to travel to be near the child. These actions violate numerous professional obligations to provide medical care that is grounded on the well-being of the child and the integrity of the family and to ensure that vulnerable children are protected by due process.[28] That medical associations and licensing boards have neither asserted the professional accountability of these physicians nor provided guidance to medical boards on how to investigate and penalize physicians for drugging, restraining, or transferring children to sites not known by their families is a failure to leverage physician accountability to improve the treatment of the children or increase the transparency of these centers.

## A Brief History and Overview of Torture

The word *torture* comes from the Latin *torques*, "twist," perhaps referring to the common technique of distorting a victim's joints or torso to cause pain. Twelfth-century French officials used it as a noun, i.e., applying "the torture" to extract confessions or testimony. Four hundred years later, the noun had crossed to England. In 1591 William Shakespeare used *torture* as a verb throughout *Henry VI*. Two hundred years ago, three-fourths of the world's people were slaves or serfs

who were subject to peremptory torture.[29] The Roman Catholic Church was torturing when it banned Cesare Beccaria's 1764 essay against torture, an Enlightenment work that spoke for a European abolitionist movement.[30] By 1850 European
governments had largely abandoned legal torture.[31] Christian churches followed
suit. Islamic courts are the last religious authorities to impose stoning, beatings,
and amputations. The nineteenth-century abolition of slavery was a major step in
reducing torture. The prevalence and trends in torture after World War II are discussed in chapter 14. Interested readers can easily find histories describing ancient
and contemporary torture. Rejali's and Ruthven's works cited in this chapter stand
out as profound cultural critiques.

Although extrajudicial torture varies by country and culture, some practices
are nearly universal.[32] The prison is typically filthy. Toilets are a bucket, a hole, a
corner of the cell, or less often, a toilet without a seat. Soap and water for washing
are restricted; hot water is not provided. Food is dirty, boring, bug infested, and
restricted. Medical attention is rare and cursory. The imprisonment begins by iso-
lating, humiliating, and degrading the prisoner and depriving him or her of sleep.
Prisoners are often kept nude and are blindfolded or held in the dark to increase
their fear and sense of vulnerability. Sometimes bright lights and loud sounds
are used to overwhelm senses and ensure sleeplessness. Nearly all prisoners are
exposed to heat or cold. Some are hosed with cold water that is left to evaporate
in cool environments. After an initial phase of isolation and brutal interrogation,
some prisoners are moved to crowded cells.

Physical torture almost always includes beatings, sometimes with fists or trun-
cheons. Some beatings are done with whips or bamboo canes that cut flesh and
leave scars. Beating or caning or whipping is done on the buttocks, the back, the
back of the legs, and especially, the soles of the feet (a technique called "falanga,"
which produces long-lasting disability).[33] Men's genitals are routinely beaten or
kicked.[34] Slapping ears with a cuffed palm might be mockingly announced, "¡Un
teléfono para usted!" (A telephone call for you!). This can lead to lifelong hearing
loss. Blows to the head can cause a brain injury that leads to depression.[35] Beatings
with blunt or softened objects do not leave scars but do produce bruises; officials
often wait for these to disappear before a physician, relative, or human rights advocate is allowed to see a prisoner.

A variety of abuses are less regularly used. Two-thirds of survivors report
being suspended by an extremity or digit or being contorted into positions in
which joints are subjected to extraordinary flexion, extension, or rotation. This can
tear ligaments, tendons, and nerves or dislocate joints.[36] Some prisoners are forced
into small boxes or cages for extended periods. Tight ligatures are sometimes
wrapped around extremities or genitalia. These can cause scars or permanent disability by interrupting the blood supply or damaging nerves. About a fourth of
victims are subjected to internal and external thermal or chemical burns by, for
example, being forced to drink acid, being burned with cigarettes or a torch, or
having caustic enemas (e.g., acids, lye, or gasoline). About a fourth of survivors

report being subjected to electric shock on the skin, under the skin, or in body cavities, including the rectum, vagina, or throat. Sometimes electric cattle prods are used to induce muscle spasms on the body or in the back of the throat. Some prisoners are given drugs that cause hallucinations, convulsions, painful muscle spasms, diarrhea, or coma-inducing low blood sugar. About 10 percent of survivors report being deprived of the ability to breath, either with a dry or wet cloth over the face or through immersion in fluid or sewage (submarino). This "water cure" differs from asphyxia-inducing waterboarding, in which prisoners are put face up, head down on a downward sloping board and then water is poured over their mouth and nose. Sometimes fluids are forced into the rectum or intestines, causing painful intestinal distention. Some regimes mutilate by pulling teeth or fingernails, cutting tongues or ears or breasts, amputating hands or feet, firing bullets into joints, or using vises to crush bones in fingers or toes. Some prisoners are castrated.

Because of shame and stigmatization, the prevalence of sexual torture is difficult to assess. About 10 percent of male survivors report being sexually abused (this figure does not include the nearly universal beating of men's genitals).[37] Of these, half report threats of castration or rape; one-third are raped or forced to perform sex on or in view of others; and one-tenth report genital electrical shocks or mutilation. Although fewer women than men are tortured, about half of women survivors report sexual torture, usually rape, sometimes in front of family members and often in the presence of other guards or soldiers.[38] Persons raped during torture often suffer severe PTSD and sexual dysfunction after their release.[39] Forty to seventy percent of torture survivors develop PTSD; anxiety disorders; depression; cognitive deficits, such as difficulty concentrating or learning; chronic pain; or somatoform disorders (e.g., chronic stomach pain).[40]

Psychological torture entails subjecting persons to extreme fear (e.g., by threatening them or their loved ones, forcing them to witness sham executions, causing asphyxia, or forcing them to watch or hear another prisoner being tortured). It also includes humiliation (e.g., forcing nudity, forcing a person to pose for pornography and telling him or her it will be made public, forcing a person to wear the underwear of the opposite sex), degradation, and stress (e.g., loud sounds or bright lights). It can further include being forced to abuse another prisoner or being subjected to prolonged social isolation, sensory deprivation, solitary confinement, or sleep deprivation.[41] Some prisoners are forced to witness the rape, torture, or murder of a loved one.

Although physical torture always entails psychological abuse, some regimes argue that "pure" psychological abuse is not really torture. The claim is false. First, the fear associated with being subjected to a sham execution causes physical stress that can result in heart attack, stroke, or death.[42] From the victim's point of view, being subjected to sham executions or being put in a grave with a corpse or in a rat-infested latrine pit can be as terrifying as being beaten. Second, psychological torture is as likely as physical torture to cause PTSD.[43] Third, it is impossible for a torturer to predict which prisoners will be able to psychically or physically survive torture without death or injury or without acquiring a fatal mental illness. Rates of PTSD and depression after torture are not predictable from prisoner to prisoner according to the severity of technique applied or according to whether a person has predominantly psychological rather than physical torture. Finally, the consequences of psychological torture can damage a victim's familial, personal, and community identity.[44]

Torture is a holistic abuse. Prisoners are always subjected to multiple, simultaneous, and sequenced techniques, and they endure them with varying and poorly understood capacities for resilience. There is no scientific grounding for an argument that there is minimally harmful torture.

## Torture for Interrogation

There are two major theories of how coercion might assist interrogation. Pain interrogation posits that people will tell the truth in order to stop pain to themselves or someone they care about. Psychiatric regression interrogation (also called learned helplessness interrogation) tries to make prisoners so psychologically dependent on the interrogator that they become truthful. In both methods, interrogators do not want the interrogatee to become so injured or psychotic as to be unable to give information. Research shows both approaches to be ineffective.[45]

The CIA's Clandestine Services department sponsored eleven years of research on interrogation in Project MK-Ultra during the Cold War.[46] When MK-Ultra ended in 1964, the CIA continued the research under Project MK-Search for another decade. These studies aimed to (1) develop ways to train American personnel to resist coercive interrogation and (2) determine whether it was possible that the Soviets, Koreans, or Chinese could brainwash prisoners along the lines of Richard Condon's 1959 potboiler *The Manchurian Candidate*, in which a prisoner of war (POW) was programmed to assassinate a US presidential candidate. CIA-funded researchers studied Korean, Chinese, and Soviet interrogation methods in more than two hundred experiments employing hypnosis, stress, electric shock, coma, sensory deprivation, sedatives, hallucinogens, or drugs to create the symptoms of diseases or disabilities. Although the CIA destroyed its research papers, its director, Richard Helms, testified to Congress that both studies had been unproductive. A declassified CIA *Counterintelligence Interrogation Manual* from 1963 refers to MK-Ultra's findings:

> The threat of death has often been found to be worse than useless. . . . No report of scientific investigation on the effect of debility upon the interrogatee's power of resistance has been discovered. For centuries, interrogators have employed various methods of inducing physical weakness, prolonged constraint; prolonged exertion, extremes of heat, cold or moisture; and deprivation or drastic reduction of food or sleep. Apparently, the assumption is

that lowering the source's physical resistance will lower his psychological capacity for opposition. . . . Prolonged exertion, loss of sleep, etc., themselves become patterns to which the subject adjusts through apathy. . . . Interrogatees who are withholding but who feel qualms of guilt and a secret desire to yield are likely to become intractable if made to endure pain.[47]

The 1983 CIA *Human Resource Exploitation Manual* came to the same conclusion: "Use of force is a poor technique. . . . However, the use of force is not to be confused with psychological ploys, verbal trickery, or other nonviolent and non-coercive ruses."[48] The Army's *Interrogation Field Manual* of 1987 reiterated the same conclusions.[49]

The governments of Nazi Germany, China, North Vietnam, the United Kingdom, and Israel all found pain to be an unreliable interrogation technique. As prisoners disintegrate, harden, or dissociate under pain, they tend to give inaccurate, useless, or misleading information.[50] Although American POWs subjected to psychiatric stress by Korean, Chinese, or the Soviet captors seemed to be more willing to make anti-American statements while in captivity than those who were tortured with pain, there is no evidence that psychological torture improved the ability of those enemy regimes to get truth from those prisoners.[51] During the war on terror, Secretary of Defense Donald Rumsfeld's advisers also cited research showing the inefficacy of harsh interrogation.[52]

The National Defense Intelligence College has conducted the most recent large-scale review of interrogation methods. This rich historical, theoretical, and scientific review notes, among many other things, "research indicates that a perception of coercion can negatively affect the tenor of the relationship between the educer and the source and decrease the likelihood that the source will comply or cooperate."[53]

In addition to being ineffective, torture is counterproductive:

1.  Inaccurate information elicited by pain stresses the limited analytic capacity of intelligence agencies. In this way the information acquired through coercive interrogation makes it more, not less, difficult for analysts to find valuable, actionable intelligence. False intelligence can lead to misguided government policies or to needless (and dangerous) missions. As the CIA's 1963 *KUBARK* manual put it, "Pain is quite likely to produce false confessions, concocted as a means of escaping from distress. Time-consuming delay results, while investigation is conducted and the admissions are proven untrue."[54]

2.  Torture diminishes the possibility of reverting to effective interrogation methods, such as building rapport, finding common interests, exploiting a subject's jealousy of comrades, and arriving at agreements in which prisoners come to see telling the truth as being in their best interest. Interrogators who abuse prisoners also risk forfeiting their own emotional equanimity, which is necessary for effective interrogation.[55]

3. Torture alienates persons who might be recruited to become informants. The CIA's 1983 *Human Resource Exploitation Manual* states, "Use of force . . . may damage subsequent collection efforts."[56] Many Federal Bureau of Investigation (FBI) reports of interrogations during the war on terror tell of prisoners who refused to cooperate with interrogators because of harsh, abusive, or degrading treatment they meted out.

4. Torture tends to harden the prisoner's political commitment and perception of the evil of the interrogating authority. Some prisoners experience torture as validating their self-importance, the rightness of their cause, or conversely, the evil of the torturing side. For example, some Palestinian prisoners tortured by Israelis considered the torture a rite of passage that bonded them to their cause, confirmed the evil of Israel, and proved their trustworthiness to comrades.[57]

5. Coercive interrogation is ill suited to asymmetrical warfare between a regular army and indigenous guerrillas who live among a large sympathetic population. Terrorist profiling by the regular army cannot identify the key persons in the communities where guerrillas live.[58] Hundreds of citizens have bits of knowledge. Dragnets for coercive interrogation are expensive and ineffective. Proponents of interrogational torture sometimes cite unvalidated accounts of French soldiers who successfully used torture to learn about terrorist attacks during Algeria's war for independence from France.[59] Those abuses and the difficult-to-confirm successes alienated the Algerian population and fueled the resistance; France lost the war. A similar pattern unfolded in Iraq, where the release of the photographs of prisoner torture in Abu Ghraib prison was followed by a drop in Iraqi support for US forces from 63 percent to 9 percent.[60]

6. Abusive interrogation can foster an "arms race" between interrogators and prisoners. Targeted groups learn the techniques that will be used against their members and then prepare their colleagues accordingly. They take measures to limit the amount of damaging information that any individual can disclose.

7. Torture might increase the duration and casualties of war by causing potentially tortured adversaries to fight longer to avoid torture and capture.

8. Secretary of State Gen. Colin Powell and his chief legal adviser, Howard Taft IV, argued that torture invites retaliatory torture and encourages dictators to justify their own use of torture with the excuse that leading human rights nations torture.[61]

9. Evidence obtained by torture is often inadmissible at trial.[62] The inadmissibility of that evidence is part of why the CIA dissociated itself from harsh interrogations.[63]

10. Torture damages the military, intelligence institutions, and their personnel. The CIA's *Human Resource Exploitation Manual* asserts, "Torture lowers the moral caliber of the organization that uses it and corrupts those that rely on it as the quick and easy way out." In 2003 Defense Secretary Rumsfeld's Working Group on Detainee Interrogations warned him, "Participation by US military personnel in interrogations which use techniques that are more aggressive than those appropriate for POWs would constitute a significant departure from traditional US military norms and could have an adverse impact on the cultural self-image of US military forces."[64] It harms unit cohesion and esprit de corps.[65] Torture psychologically traumatizes the soldiers who perform it. Soldiers who passively witness or who commit atrocities suffer more severe PTSD than those who kill during combat.[66]

11. Torture creates the possibility of prosecution of the torturers or their leaders after the torturing regime loses power.

The ticking time bomb argument is a hypothetical scenario crafted to support the moral case for torture. Interestingly, in 1879 Fyodor Dostoevsky wrote a version of the argument in *The Brothers Karamazov*. Ivan poses this question to his younger brother, a priest: "Imagine that you are creating a fabric of human destiny with the object of making men happy in the end, giving them peace and rest at last, but that it was essential and inevitable to torture to death only one tiny creature—that baby beating its breast with its fist, for instance—and to found that edifice on its unavenged tears, would you consent to be the architect on those conditions?"[67] Ivan's hypothetical argument was constructed to compel Ayosha to accept the utilitarian conclusion that if an innocent baby could be tortured for the social good, then it was certainly permissible to torture criminals who were a threat to society. The ticking time bomb argument is similarly crafted: If an enemy might have knowledge of an impending attack, then it is permissible to torture that person to get the intelligence needed to prevent that attack. Popular fiction, such as the television series *24*, which ran during the war on terror, presents a seductive case for the ticking time bomb argument as digital clocks count down while frantic government agents work to prevent innocent people from doom. To its adherents, the ticking time bomb argument means that it is idealistic and irresponsible to ban torture.[68] The argument fails in that it presumes that interrogational torture is productive, ignoring the research showing that coercion is ineffective and counterproductive.

Coercive interrogations under the ticking time bomb argument are still ethically problematic. First, what degree of certainty about a prisoner's specific knowledge is required to justify the extreme act of interrogational torture? Can an intelligence agency use the ticking time bomb argument to justify the torture of any person allegedly affiliated with a criminal enterprise on the assumption that he or she might possess knowledge that could help avert a crime? A related corollary is, Is it moral to use interrogational torture knowing that most of those questioned will be either innocent or ignorant of actionable intelligence? If so, what does society owe the many innocent victims of torture? How can they or their families possibly be compensated? Second, is it moral to torture an enemy who is unlikely to give useful information despite being tortured? On a related note, is it moral to torture that person's spouse or child if that is the only way to get information? Third, what are the thresholds for the degree of damage of the attack to be prevented? Is it justifiable to torture to save one person, ten, a thousand, a city? Fourth, does the ticking time bomb argument require a clock? That is, should interrogational torture be limited to situations in which evidence points to an imminent attack, or can it be used in the situation of an inchoate or long-range fear of possible attack? In real world intelligence gathering, even if a prisoner knows something about a future crime, that piece of intelligence is by itself rarely of immediate utility. Analysts must fit the prisoner's knowledge into a larger set of information, a process that usually takes a considerable amount of time.

Some propose procedural safeguards (such as torture warrants) in which a court would weigh the gravity or probability of the crime that interrogational torture would endeavor to prevent.[69] Some suggest that torture should remain illegal but that courts should allow an after-the-fact "necessity" defense, somewhat akin to allowing a person to claim the necessity of murder in self-defense. History does not justify confidence in such measures. Regimes that torture have always spread the practice far beyond the narrow justifications of the popular fictional images of ticking time bomb scenarios as they abuse a widening circle of innocent persons and ignorant opponents. As the Association for the Prevention of Torture argues in a comprehensive monograph, accepting the ticking bomb argument lights a fuse on a human rights bomb in civil societies.[70]

# 4

# WHAT IS A
# TORTURE DOCTOR?

The question, What is a torture doctor? invites a useless tautology: "A torture doctor is a doctor who tortures." The tautology clarifies nothing. It fails because a torture doctor is a sphinx, a human face with a lion's body. The torture doctor is a chimera of beast and healer—the immorality of torture and the moral profession of medicine. Defining a torture doctor requires understanding how those two parts make a distinctive whole.

The definition begins by inspecting the moral core of medicine. The Hippocratic precept "Do not harm" comes to mind.[1] Torture harms. Torture violates respect for the health and choices of the prisoner. The preface to the WMA's 1975 Declaration of Tokyo says, "It is the privilege of the physician to practice medicine in the service of humanity, to preserve and restore bodily and mental health without distinction as to persons, and to comfort and to ease the suffering of his or her patients."[2] The United Nations' Principles of Medical Ethics Relevant to the Role of Health Personnel, particularly Physicians, in the Protection of Prisoners and Detainees against Torture and Other Cruel, Inhuman or Degrading Treatment or Punishment blends the moral foundation with law: "It is a gross contravention of medical ethics, as well as an offence under applicable international instruments, for health personnel, particularly physicians, to engage, actively or passively, in acts which constitute participation in, complicity in, incitement to or attempts to commit torture or other cruel, inhuman or degrading treatment or punishment."[3]

In addition to being bound to the moral duty to heal, physicians are accountable to science. A physician who promotes almond extracts as a cure for cancer has abandoned science and thus the claim to medical excellence. Torture may appropriate the garb of science to claim authority, but it is at its core antiscientific. Nazi "race hygiene" was a false science created to justify segregation and genocide. The Soviets' spurious concept of "sluggish schizophrenia" was created to justify imprisoning dissidents, invalidating their political beliefs as signs of mental illness, and to impose brutal abuse with drugs (see chapter 6). US intelligence agencies' research had discredited the idea that coercion would facilitate interrogation long before those same agencies lifted up the gobbledygook of "learned helplessness" to empower behavioral science consultation teams (BSCTs) to brutalize war on terror prisoners (see chapters 3 and 13).

The chaotic advice in torture manuals reveals the unscientific nature of torture.[4] Some manuals advise escalating harshness quickly; others say build slowly. Some say that a prisoner should never hear or see other tortured prisoners; others say that prisoners should hear fellow prisoners crying out in pain at the earliest opportunity. Lacking a scientific foundation, torture evolves from contrivance and imitation. Its regional variants are based on teaching by sponsors, local traditions, and available materials.

Finally, a medical license is a prerequisite for a torture doctor. In one sense it certifies that the practitioner has medical knowledge and skills. But torturing governments are not much interested in clinical finesse in the healing sciences. Torture is about power. The medical license comes with the authority to write official medical documents (e.g., death certificates and other medical records) and to access and order the use of certain drugs. The torture doctor puts these powers in the service of torture. For example, the knowledge of a painful side effect and the authority to prescribe it, both of which would suggest prudence and caution to a healer, become tools for the torture doctor. The authority to create official medical records and death certificates is a power for concealing torture. It is difficult to overturn a death certificate that falsely records that a prisoner died of a heart attack. Ironically, the medical license brings torture doctors within the ambit of special forms of accountability, boards that grant licenses, clinical facilities that grant practice privileges, and medical associations that are a source of prestige and collegiality after the torture career ends. These bodies, as we will see in part 3, sometimes hold torture doctors accountable for violating the duties of a medical career.

The 1975 version of the Declaration of Tokyo proposes four ways to assess a physician's complicity with torture:

> The doctor shall not provide any premises, instruments, substances or knowledge to facilitate the practice of torture . . . or to diminish the ability of the victim to resist such treatment.
>
> The doctor shall not be present during any procedure during which torture . . . [is] used or threatened.
>
> A doctor must have complete clinical independence in deciding upon the care of a person for whom he or she is medically responsible. The doctor's fundamental role is to alleviate the distress of his or her fellow men, and no motive whether personal, collective or political shall prevail against this higher purpose.

Where a prisoner refuses nourishment and is considered by the doctor as capable of forming an unimpaired and rational judgment concerning the consequences of such voluntary refusal of nourishment, he or she shall not be fed artificially.

Some argue that terms like *countenance, condone, complete clinical independence,* and *complicity in* are too vague for the weighty task of judging and punishing torture doctors. They argue that a torture doctor should be judged by a set of specified behaviors.[5] That behavioral definition of medical torture would set aside the tricky problem of assessing the physician against the ethos of the medical profession.[6] It would be as clear and fair as a speed limit. As we shall see in part 3, the probable increase in accountability from such a behavioral approach would be small given that it does not address the critical lack of will to hold torture doctors accountable.

It is, however, possible to develop a taxonomy of torture doctoring that is more specific than the list in the Declaration of Tokyo. This taxonomy would assess the clinician in two categories of transgressions: (1) misuse of medical skills and knowledge and (2) misuse of the authorities or duties conferred by a medical license. Table 4.1 proposes the first tier of subcategories under these categories.

**TABLE 4.1**  Taxonomy of torture doctoring

A.  Misuse of medical knowledge or skills
  1.  The physician inflicts torture.
  2.  The physician misuses medical knowledge or skills to abet torture by others.
  3.  The physician misuses medical skills while providing treatment.
  4.  The physician misuses medical knowledge and skills to clear prisoners as fit for torture.
  5.  The physician misuses medical knowledge or skills to monitor prisoners being tortured so that the torture may proceed.
  6.  Miscellaneous

B.  Misuse of the authorities or duties conferred by a medical license
  1.  The physician misuses the authority to acquire and release medical materials for the purpose of torture.
  2.  The physician fails to create accurate medical records in order to abet torture.
  3.  The physician fails to undertake the treatment of a tortured person in a manner that abets the abuse.
  4.  The physician fails to safeguard medical records for the tortured prisoners to use for their own interests.
  5.  The physician fails to report torture.
  6.  The physician abets abusive research on prisoners that violates established research standards.
  7.  Miscellaneous

The appendix at the end of this book gives case examples of what might fall within these categories. Several cautions on the anecdotes in the appendix (as well as throughout this book) must be made. First, I name countries to illustrate the diversity of nations where torture doctors work; similar actions are seen in many other nations. Second, the cited behaviors oversample open societies, where human rights reporting is possible. Closed societies, like Syria, Burma, the People's Republic of China, or North Korea, are very difficult to investigate. The myriad of subcategories in table 4.1 and of behaviors cited in the appendix show the difficulty of creating a behavioral definition of torture doctoring. Finally, the behaviors tabulated in this book are not an exhaustive compilation of torture doctors' work.

I do not believe that a simple list of behaviors that constitute torture doctoring can be crafted. Torturers are creative. If abusively loud sounds are barred, inaudible hypersonic noise will be introduced. If complicity with methods that leave scars is to be the definitive evidence of physician collaboration with torture, regimes will shift to methods, such as waterboarding, that do not leave scars, that is, to techniques Rejali calls "stealth torture."[7] Thus, each newly minted technique will set off a new cycle of debating the behavioral definition. Finally, torture uses multiple techniques in various sequences against persons of various debilities and resilience. Even if all the individual elements of a program of torture did not include any of a list of banned behaviors, the total, multicomponent regimen of torture could well remain deeply traumatizing.

This chapter began with a question: What is a torture doctor? I propose the following definition:

Torture doctor—A licensed physician who directly or indirectly puts (a) medical knowledge or skills or (b) the authorities, duties, or privileges conferred by the medical license in the service of "torture" or "cruel, inhuman, or degrading treatment or punishment" as such terms are understood in international law.

# PART II

A TIME OF IMPUNITY

# 5

# JUDGING THE NAZI DOCTORS

The foundation for trying Nazi leaders for their war crimes was laid before World War II ended. After their failure to take Stalingrad, retreating Germans murdered civilians with ferocious intensity. In October 1943 US president Franklin Delano Roosevelt, British prime minister Winston Churchill, and Soviet general secretary of the Central Committee of the Communist Party Joseph Stalin signed the Moscow Declaration on German Atrocities, promising that those who had shed "innocent blood" would be pursued "to the uttermost ends of the earth . . . in order that justice may be done."[1] The Allies knew of the Nazi concentration camps, although they did not grasp their stupendous scale or purpose.

Ten months after D-Day, the Fourth Armored Division of the Eighty-Ninth Infantry came across the Nazi Ohrdruf labor camp, where 11,700 starving, enslaved prisoners were being worked to death to build a railroad. The soldiers were so horrified at what they saw that they notified Gen. Dwight Eisenhower, the Supreme Allied Commander. He promptly visited the camp and cabled Washington on April 15, 1945, just eleven days after the camp was discovered:

> The things I saw beggar description. . . . The visual evidence and the verbal testimony of starvation, cruelty and bestiality were so overpowering as to leave me a bit sick. In one room, where they were piled up twenty or thirty naked men, killed by starvation, George Patton would not even enter. He said that he would get sick if he did so. I made the visit deliberately, in order to be in a position to give first-hand evidence of these things if ever, in the future, there develops a tendency to charge these allegations merely to "propaganda."[2]

General Eisenhower soon learned that the Ohrdruf camp was a satellite of Buchenwald concentration camp, thirty miles away. Buchenwald, in turn,

35

belonged to a galaxy of about twenty thousand Nazi prison camps. Eisenhower did not know that doctors played major roles in the Nazi death machine.[3] Jews and others from as far away as Cos, the tiny Greek island where Hippocrates had founded his medical school, had been rounded up and sent to the Nazi concentration camps, where physicians selected millions to be put to slave labor and culled the weakest for murder.[4] The Nazi medical profession was garbed in the pseudoscience of race hygiene, which rationalized race classifications, segregation, sterilizations, murder of the ill, and genocide of "lesser races." In the course of this slaughter, doomed prisoners were selected to be the subjects for cruel research.

World War II showed the world that doctors could commit medical war crimes. It was a physician, Capt. John W. Thompson, who identified distinctive acts as medical war crimes, or, as he first saw them, lethal experiments on prisoners.[5] Thompson was a bilingual psychiatrist, an empathic clinician, an experienced medical researcher, and a broadly read, somewhat ascetic humanist. In May 1945 Thompson was deployed to Bergen-Belsen concentration camp to help demobilize the camp. Thirteen thousand survivors died after the liberation of the camp, mostly because of the combined effects of starvation and typhus. Many prisoners were profoundly mentally ill with PTSD, anxiety disorders, psychosomatic pain, and depression.

In September 1945 Thompson was again transferred to analyze intelligence about the value of Nazi science. He thought physicians should be held accountable for committing medical crimes on behalf of the state. His insight came from reviewing a study of night vision, in which a Nazi physiologist, Gotthilft von Studnitz, had injected prisoners' eyes to dilate the irises and then had the prisoners murdered so he could remove the eyes for study. Thompson was horrified that an experiment was predicated on murdering its subjects. By November 1945 he had compiled many such studies and wrote a memo asserting that Nazi physicians had free rein to conduct experiments and proposing the term *medical war crimes*. Ultimately, it was learned that Nazi doctors had infected prisoners with typhus, spotted fever, hepatitis, and tuberculosis. They tested lethal doses of poison, did surgery without anesthesia, burned people with phosphorus, cut off limbs for crude transplants, and subjected people to lethal cold or lack of oxygen. After researching the cheapest way to kill people, physicians selected chronically ill persons or those who were exhausted by prison labor to be murdered.

Thompson's concept of a medical war crime led to the creation of the International Scientific Commission for the Investigation of Medical War Crimes, which convened a panel of physicians to review Nazi experiments that Thompson and others had discovered. The commission's finding that the studies were cruel and without merit was the cornerstone for a criminal trial of Nazi doctors.[6] Thompson's discovery of medical war crimes obsessed him, seared him, and enabled him to profoundly mark history.

# The Nazi Doctors' Trial at Nuremberg

In 1935 the Nazi Party announced its infamous race laws at a huge rally in Nuremberg. After the war Nuremberg had a courthouse and a hotel that had not been totally destroyed by Allied bombs. As Thompson was drafting his memo on medical war crimes, the Allies were going through the task of organizing the International Military Tribunal to try Nazi leaders, as promised by the Moscow Declaration on German Atrocities.[7] Most of those leaders were sent to prison or executed. After the International Military Tribunal, the United States oversaw twelve trials of war criminals before the Nuremberg Military Tribunals. The defendants were roughly grouped by occupation (e.g., medicine, law, industry, field commanders, government ministers) Thompson's ardent and extensively documented work ensured that doctors were tried first.

*United States of America v. Karl Brandt, et al.* (the Nazi doctors' trial) ran from December 1946 until August 1947.[8] The defendants included twenty physicians and three men with scientific or medical oversight duties. The number of defendants was prescribed by the size of the box for seating them. At the end seven were sentenced to death, nine were given prison terms, and seven were acquitted. Brig. Gen. Telford Taylor, a bilingual American lawyer, gave the opening address. He spoke of the right to try war criminals and on four themes in the indictment: (1) the criminal conspiracy on Nazi murders, (2) the cruelty of Nazi research, (3) the lack of consent by victims of Nazi medical experiments, and (4) the lack of scientific merit to the death camp experiments. He brought together medical ethics and war crimes in his address to the court, and his remarks merit an extensive quotation:

> I intend to pass very briefly over matters of medical ethics, such as the conditions under which a physician may lawfully perform a medical experiment upon a person who has voluntarily subjected himself to it, or whether experiments may lawfully be performed upon criminals who have been condemned to death. This case does not present such problems. No refined questions confront us here.
>
> None of the victims of the atrocities perpetrated by these defendants were volunteers, and this is true regardless of what these unfortunate people may have said or signed before their tortures began. . . .
>
> Whatever book or treatise on medical ethics we may examine, and whatever expert on forensic medicine we may question, will say that it is a fundamental and inescapable obligation of every physician under any known system of law not to perform a dangerous experiment without the subject's consent. In the tyranny that was Nazi Germany, no one could give such a consent to the medical agents of the State; everyone lived in fear and acted under duress. . . . Were it necessary, one could make a long list of the respects in which the experiments which these defendants performed departed from every known standard of medical ethics. But the gulf between these atrocities

and serious research in the healing art is so patent that such a tabulation would be cynical.

If the principles announced in the [German law for protecting animals from inhumane experiments] had been followed for human beings as well, this indictment would never have been filed. It is perhaps the deepest shame of the defendants that it probably never even occurred to them that human beings should be treated with at least equal humanity.

This case is one of the simplest and clearest of those that will be tried in this building. It is also one of the most important. It is true that the defendants in the box were not among the highest leaders of the Third Reich. . . . The things that these defendants did, like so many other things that happened under the Third Reich, were the result of the noxious merger of German militarism and Nazi racial objectives. We will see the results of this merger in many other fields of German life; we see it here in the field of medicine. . . .

The fact that these investigators had free and unrestricted access to human beings to be experimented upon misled them to the dangerous and fallacious conclusion that the results would thus be better and more quickly obtainable than if they had gone through the labor of preparation, thinking and meticulous pre-investigation. . . .

Who could German medicine look to to keep the profession true to its traditions and protect it from the ravaging inroads of Nazi pseudo-science? This was the supreme responsibility of the leaders of German medicine—men like Rostock and Rose and Schroeder and Handloser [defendants]. That is why their guilt is greater than that of any of the other defendants in the dock. They are the men who utterly failed their country and their profession, who showed neither courage nor wisdom nor the vestiges of moral character.[9]

Taylor did not mention Hippocrates or "do no harm." He did not propose that medical ethics is the same during wartime as it is during peace or the same for prisoners as it is for free persons. German doctors oversaw the murders of seventy thousand disabled children and adults and millions more in camps. But as far as medical ethics goes, aside from a passing reference to race hygiene, the prosecutor focused on a person's right to consent to or refuse being subjected to a dangerous experiment.

Medical ethics had a hard time at Nuremberg. Dr. Andrew Ivy, a celebrity US doctor, pushed his political connections to get the American Medical Association to send him to testify as an expert witness. He presented an American code of ethics as the standard of care to guide research with prisoners. Under cross-examination he revealed that he wrote the code for the Nuremberg trial *after* learning of the Nazi medical war crimes.[10] To make matters worse, Ivy recognized the central point of the Hippocratic oath (i.e., that medicine must have a moral core) but said that it applied only to a doctor-patient relationship and not to the relationship between a doctor and a research subject, which was the ethics issue of the trial.[11] Dr. Werner Liebrand, a German physician expert witness, disagreed with Ivy's distinction between clinical and research ethics: "The morality of a physician is to hold back his natural research urge which may result in doing harm, in order to maintain his basic medical attitude that is laid down in the Oath of Hippocrates."[12]

Dr. Leo Alexander, a Jewish physician who had emigrated from Austria to the United States in 1933, was Taylor's chief medical adviser. During the trial he was bound to discretion and did not openly speak to the core conflict between Nazi medicine and medical ethics other than claiming that the "Hippocratic attitude" prohibits lethal experiments.[13] After the trial, when he was at liberty to speak on the lessons of Nazi medicine, he concluded that the totalitarian Nazi ideology of race hygiene had led physicians to submerge their professional duties to individual patients to serve the false view of a healthy race.[14] He contrasted the cowardice of Nazi physicians with the heroism of Dutch physicians who at great peril refused to cooperate with the Nazi search for Jews.[15]

The Nuremberg trials missed an opportunity to discuss how medical ethics addressed the Nazi clinical practice as an evil or racist medical ideology. The Hippocratic oath is written in the first person to emphasize personal accountability. These three passages are as germane to defining the rotten core of Nazi medicine as they are to assessing torture doctors:

> I will use regimens for the benefit of the ill in accordance with my ability and my judgment, but from what is to their harm or injustice I will keep them. . . .
>
> I will not give a drug that is deadly to anyone if asked, nor will I suggest the way to such a counsel [in the Hippocratic era, this passage referred to refraining from the widespread murder and assassination intrigues of the day]. . . .
>
> Into as many houses as I may enter, I will go for the benefit of the ill, while being far from all voluntary and destructive injustice, especially from sexual acts both upon women's bodies and upon men's, both of the free and of the slaves ["slaves" aptly describes prisoners].[16]

With medical ethics at the Nazi doctors' trial confined to the issue of the uncoerced consent of a research subject and Dr. Ivy's botched testimony, the prosecution prudently turned to consider criminal acts. To be fair, medical ethics was simply not prepared to address anything like the evil of Nazi medicine. Alexander, Thompson, and Ivy crafted the Nuremberg Code of Ethics for Medical Research, which the court revised and included among its records. Although the code's ten principles became a foundation for modern research ethics, the trial transcript shows that the Nazi physicians were convicted for war crimes like murder and criminal conspiracy rather than for violations of medical ethics. As a judge put it during the trial:

Of the ten principles [in the Nuremberg Code] which have been enumerated, our judicial concern, of course, is with those requirements which are
purely legal in nature—or which at least are so clearly related to matters legal
that they assist us in determining criminal culpability and punishment. To go
beyond that point would lead us into a field that would be beyond our sphere
of competence. . . .

Obviously all of these experiments involving brutalities, tortures, disabling
injury, and death were performed in complete disregard of international conventions, the laws and customs of war, the general principles of criminal law
as derived from the criminal laws of all civilized nations, and Control Council
Law No. 10 [a document setting the framework for the Nuremberg trials].
Manifestly human experiments under such conditions are contrary to the
principles of the law of nations as they result from usages established among
civilized peoples from the laws of humanity and from the dictates of public
conscience.[17]

In other words the Nuremberg court centered on the crimes committed by
the Nazi doctors rather than on their medical ethics. Lawyer James McHaney's
seventy-eight-page closing argument on July 14, 1947, made only passing reference to medical ethics: "A distinguished American scientist [Ivy] said in this
court, 'There is no state or politician under the sun who could force me to perform a medical experiment which I thought was morally unjustified.'"[18] Despite
the limited role of medical ethics, the Nazi doctors' trial was an unprecedented
act of creative justice. The occupational clustering of defendants in the series of
trials created a critical mass of doctors and medical images that forced the public
and the profession to recognize the special issue raised by physicians committing
human rights crimes for their governments. The profession's first response took
place in Paris a month after the trial adjourned.

## Paris and Geneva

In 1947 Paris was a city recovering from war. Telephone and electrical service was
erratic. The Crillon Hotel managed to get its central heating working and became
a prized destination for visiting Americans. Art that had been hidden from the
Nazis was coming out of barns, basements, wine cellars, and nunneries. The
golden age of haute couture was born. Eva Perón was dressing up. Henri Matisse
was in bed with scissors creating his jazz collages. Édith Piaf was France's war-
bling diva. Laurel and Hardy were performing at cabarets. Georges Bizet's *Sym-
phony in C* had its world's premiere at the National Opera. James Baldwin was
staying at the Hotel Verneuil; its only virtue was that it was inexpensive. Simone
de Beauvoir signed the Proclamation for International Women's Day in honor of
women who fought tyranny. Survivors from Jewish families were unsuccessfully
trying to retrieve their stolen wealth from banks. Bitter recriminations about Nazi

collaboration were ripping society apart. Jean Paul Sartre was writing a play titled *Dirty Hands.*

On September 17, 1947, delegates from twenty-six national medical associations made a pilgrimage to liberated Paris to convene the first General Assembly of an organization that they would call the World Medical Association.[19] It is remarkable that the WMA managed to convene at all. Europe was smoldering. Funds were scarce. Health care infrastructures around the world had suffered enormous damage and were inundated with casualties, demobilized veterans, refugees, and malnourished civilians with enormous untended needs. Most of the delegations came from Europe. Canada and the United States sent the only Western Hemisphere delegations. Delegates from China, India, Arab Palestine, the future Israel, and Turkey came from Asia. South Africa sent the only African delegation. The Soviet Union did not participate; Poland and Czech medical associations would be gone in a year.

In 1948 the WMA held its Second General Assembly in Geneva and issued an extraordinary bulletin.[20] In contrast to the Nuremberg Code of Ethics' focus on medical research, the WMA's bulletin spoke to the broader ethics issues raised by Nazi medical crimes. The WMA condemned the "betrayal of medicine" by the Nuremberg defendants and other, unindicted Nazi "doctors who carried out inhuman orders, who acted as technicians, or who connived at criminal acts." Their crimes included preparing means of bacterial warfare and placing "their medical knowledge at the disposal of others concerned with such warfare." The WMA bulletin asserted that such doctors were personally responsible and therefore that individual punishments were necessary to deter such acts in the future: "These crimes . . . now belong to history, and the doctors of the world, having expressed their indignation, must now consider how any repetition may be prevented." It called on the German medical associations to promise, "We undertake to expel from our organization those members who have been personally guilty of the crimes referred to above." In Germany expelling a doctor had the effect of revoking his or her license to practice medicine. The WMA also endorsed criminal "judicial punishment of such crimes." That seminal WMA bulletin, which represented the WMA position arguing for personal accountability for torture doctors, is available only in academic libraries. By contrast the WMA's numerous antitorture proclamations that are silent on accountability are prominently carried on its website (see chapter 10).

The Medical Chambers of Western Germany sent a letter to the WMA. The German organization condemned "all crimes against humanity" and "all the German Physicians who had participated in the war crimes against humanity." It went on, "The [Nuremberg] trial also served to demonstrate the danger of interference of government authorities in medicine, since bureaucracies have no contact with the problems of doctors in their relationship with their patients. It was the NSDAP [National Socialist German Workers' Party, i.e., the Nazi Party] and the army that tried to interfere with the freedom of the medical profession and to destroy it."

By framing Nazi medical crimes as a collective responsibility—one caused by the Nazi government—the Medical Chambers of Western Germany rejected punishing individual Nazi physicians.

In 1948 the WMA adopted the Declaration of Geneva. Like the Hippocratic oath, the declaration was written in the first person—the voice of personal responsibility. Its rejection of Nazi medicine can be heard throughout, especially in these passages:

> I SOLEMNLY PLEDGE to consecrate my life to the service of humanity. . . .
> THE HEALTH AND LIFE OF MY PATIENT will be my first consideration. . . .
> I WILL NOT PERMIT considerations of religion, nationality, race, party politics or social standing to intervene between my duty and my patient;
> I WILL MAINTAIN the utmost respect for human life, from the time of its conception, even under threat, I will not use my medical knowledge contrary to the laws of humanity.[21]

Although the declaration does not mention torture, genocide, brutal experiments, or other specific medical war crimes, it pointedly says that doctors may not act "contrary to the laws of humanity." "Laws of humanity" was a significant phrase. The terms *international law, war crimes,* and *crimes against humanity* were all being used after World War I and the Armenian genocide of 1915. The Second and Fourth Hague Warfare Conventions of 1899 and 1907 noted the unsettled terminology: "Until a more complete code of the laws of war is issued . . . populations and belligerents remain under the protection and empire of the principles of international law, as they result from the usages established between civilized nations, from the *laws of humanity* and the requirements of the public conscience."[22] By 1948 several terms were being used to describe what we now call international law. The WMA's Declaration of Geneva was passed immediately before the newborn United Nations endorsed the Universal Declaration of Human Rights, which would assert the right to not be tortured (see chapter 8).[23] By having each physician vow in the first person to "not use my medical knowledge contrary to the laws of humanity," the WMA reiterated that individual doctors were personally bound by international law regardless of domestic laws to the contrary; "considerations of religion, nationality, race, party politics or social standing"; or "threat." Thus, up to 1948 the WMA rejected the German Medical Chambers' argument against personal responsibility for Nazi medical crimes.

The WMA did not draft procedures for its member national medical associations to hold torture doctors accountable or expel them. Instead, in 1949 it passed the International Code of Medical Ethics, asserting, "The following practices are deemed unethical: . . . Any act or advice which could weaken physical or mental resistance of a human being."[24] That language and all subsequent WMA codes and declarations are silent on holding doctors who abet crimes against humanity, including torture, accountable. The German Medical Association, now allied with the West, did not name, censure, or expel Nazi physicians who had committed war crimes. Its first president, Dr. Karl Haedekamp, was a former brown shirt and Nazi physician who spent the war implementing race policy.[25] The WMA welcomed the German Medical Association as a member in 1951.

The WMA delegates at its Paris and Geneva meetings may not have fully appreciated the implications of the political watershed that was taking place. The Nuremberg trials and the WMA's assertion of personal accountability for medical war crimes were a capstone on prosecuting medical crimes of World War II. The future belonged to the Cold War. Stalin bound the nations of Eastern Europe to the Soviet Union behind his Iron Curtain. Mao Zedong and allies established an Asian Communist bloc. For decades the Communist and Western blocs each sought to expand against, or at least contain, the other. The Cold War resulted in the consolidation of ideological, industrial, and scientific constituencies. The phrase *military-industrial complex* was coined in 1947, a year before the Declaration of Geneva and long before President Eisenhower popularized it as he left the presidency in 1961.[26]

Before the Nazi doctors' trial had even begun, the United States launched Operation Overcast in 1945, which quickly expanded from recruiting Axis aerospace experts to recruiting experts, including physicians, who worked on biochemical warfare, and it was renamed Operation Paperclip.[27] Thus, even before the WMA asserted that doctors who committed war crimes should be personally punished, Nazi medical scientists had been brought to the United States and protected from prosecution. In 1947 the British created a detention and interrogation center at the behest of the United States, called Project Dustbin, to screen scientists, mostly for Paperclip. As the political fight over which physicians to prosecute and which to recruit dragged on, enthusiasm waned for the cost and complexity of Thompson's proposal to punish Nazi doctors for war crimes.[28] In this politicized environment Thompson's passion became a liability, and he was quickly marginalized. His plan for the International Scientific Commission on the Investigation of War Crimes of a Medical Nature was deprived of funds and prosecutorial help and died.

Operation Paperclip gave impunity to several senior Nazi physicians. Dr. Hubertus Strughold, who had conducted lethal medical experiments at Dachau concentration camp, was brought to the United States to work on aerospace medicine. The details of his grotesque career were uncovered only after the "Father of Aerospace Medicine" had died in 1986.[29] Some of Strughold's colleagues (including his research assistant, Hermann Becker-Freyseng) were convicted at Nuremberg for lethal research at Dachau. Becker-Freyseng was convicted for injecting saltwater into forty prisoners and then biopsying their livers without anesthetic; all the healthy prisoners died. He was sentenced to twenty years in prison for war crimes and crimes against humanity. Paperclip promptly pulled him from prison and brought him to the United States to work on aerospace research.[30]

Paperclip also brought Drs. Kurt Blome (a senior Nazi germ warfare expert), Siegfried Ruff, and Konrad Schäfer, all of whom had been acquitted at Nuremberg, to the United States.[31] Many Nazi doctors' lives and crimes are memorialized by pathologies named after them.[32] Hugo Spatz, a Nazi neuropathologist who performed autopsies on death camp prisoners, came to the United Stated and had a distinguished career, although his name was ultimately removed from the brain disease he discovered.

The Japanese Ping Fan research facility in Manchuria was as large in area as Auschwitz-Birkenau. The Japanese military kidnapped people to use in experiments. Later, the bodies would be burned at Ping Fan's mass crematorium. Operation Paperclip recruited Japanese medical scientists who had performed lethal research on prisoners and who had created germ bombs that they tested on prisoners and communities. The Soviets captured six midlevel Japanese researchers and convicted them of war crimes. The United States referred to the Soviet trial as "propaganda."[33] The United States prevented its own war crimes investigators from seeing records detailing Japanese germ warfare experiments. The Japan Medical Association afforded impunity to its torture doctors and, with its German counterpart, was admitted to the WMA in 1951.

A story about Maj. Gen. Walter Schreiber, MD, illustrates how the impunity of doctors who had committed war crimes arises from active protection rather than from a passive failure to prosecute.[34] In 1945 Schreiber was the highest-ranking Nazi physician listed on the US Army's Central Registry of War Criminals. The Nuremberg prosecutors sought to interview him for possible charges, but the Soviet Union took him into protective custody. To the United States' surprise, the Soviets produced Schreiber at Nuremberg to testify about Nazi germ warfare. Schreiber mysteriously escaped both his Soviet handlers and the interests of Nuremberg prosecutors. The US Joint Chiefs of Staff and CIA recruited him through Operation Paperclip and brought him to work on germ warfare at an air force base in Texas. A few months after Schreiber arrived in the United States, the Boston Globe ran a headline story describing Schreiber's deadly experiments on Polish girls at Ravensbrück concentration camp. A national scandal ensued. The Joint Chiefs of Staff paid Schreiber off and put him on a boat to Argentina, where the United States helped him settle.

The Schreiber case shows how protecting a war criminal requires complex policies. A government must compile a list of officials who are to be shielded. Measures must be taken to prevent prosecutors or human rights groups from obtaining records of their crimes. Cover stories are created. Backup plans must be activated when these measures fail. As a public policy, impunity for torture policy resembles other aspects of torture policy: it is secret and subordinates truth and justice to higher national interests.

Accountability for Nazi war crimes proceeded fitfully. Although several tens of thousands of Nazi collaborators were called before trials across Europe, most of these were soldiers who raped and executed hostages and operated death camps.[35]

In the early 1950s West Germany ended denazification and enacted enormous waves of amnesties and pardons.[36] The Central Registry of War Criminals and Security Suspects still contains the names of many physicians who were never held accountable to allegations of war crimes.[37] In his opening address, Justice Robert Jackson, chief prosecution counsel for the Nuremberg tribunal, urged, "We must never forget that the record on which we judge these defendants is the record on which history will judge us tomorrow. To pass these defendants a poisoned chalice is to put it to our own lips as well."[38]

In other words, the Nuremberg verdicts do not allow a double standard. By affirming that the Nazi doctors were properly judged, we stand under the summons of the Nuremberg principles ourselves. In 1948 the WMA endorsed physician accountability for crimes against humanity. By 1949 it had gone silent on the matter. In 1951 it admitted the German and Japan Medical Associations despite the impunity that those associations afforded their doctors who had committed war crimes. The next chapters show how impunity became the rule.

# 6

# A GLOBAL MAP OF TORTURE DOCTORS

"Doctors torture with impunity." The inflection misleads. It sounds as if impunity to prosecution is an innate characteristic of torture doctors—like "Superman is invincible to bullets." The brutal truth is this: regimes promise and provide impunity to physicians who assist torture. Courts, medical licensing boards, and medical associations are actively or passively complicit with impunity by failing to develop or use procedures to hold torture doctors accountable. With impunity assured, torture doctoring has grown deep roots around the world.

There are several reasons to try to map where torture doctors practice. First, it helps assess and convey the extent of torture doctoring. Second, it identifies special strains of medically assisted torture (e.g., complicity with flogging) that may be amenable to tactically focused reforms. Third, one might hope that identifying countries with torture doctors will foster pressure on licensing boards, professional societies, and courts to hold physicians accountable. Ultimately, one might hope that the risk of exposure or accountability might increase the transparency of prisons (all of which have medical staff) and enable physicians and other human rights advocates to decrease the ferocity of torture.

It is much harder to map physician complicity with torture than it is to identify countries with torture. Beginning in 1972 Amnesty International's Campaign for the Abolition of Torture began to assess the global extent of torture. Today, the UN and hundreds of human rights organizations have taken up this task as well. In 1986 the British Medical Association (BMA) asked Amnesty how often doctors were involved in torture. Amnesty replied that "the role of doctors was usually incidental to the report on torture and it's the torture that is the focus and not the fact that doctors are involved."[1] Although the UN Special Rapporteur on Torture and human rights groups have recently been taking somewhat more care to note physicians' roles in torture, there is no indexing of such findings in their hundreds of diversely formatted reports. The only way to find such anecdotes is to tediously search each report for tiny flecks of stories. I am confident I missed hundreds of anecdotes (not counting the ones that I omitted because they were redundant) in UN reports alone. Furthermore, torturing regimes are often closed societies that obstruct prison inspections or persecute human rights advocates who might be inclined to report instances of medical complicity with torture.[2] It is, for example, nearly impossible to assess North Korea's vicious prisons. By contrast, it is possible to identify the names of at least a few prison doctors and their practices in nations with more open societies. As in the preceding chapters, I include some extended anecdotes to more fully portray the work and settings of physician collaboration with torture. Readers are advised to look at the citations in the appendix for other information on specific countries.

A map of torture doctors is a map of nations and political cultures. Boundaries are therefore messy. I crudely consider five geographic or political clusters: current and former Communist nations, West European nations outside the former Communist bloc, Asia, Africa, and Latin America. After these, I will leave geographical clusters to discuss three fairly widely practiced forms of medically assisted torture: mutilation, flogging, and medico-sexual abuse. The anecdotes occur during the interval from the Nuremberg Nazi doctors' trial until the present. The United States and the United Kingdom are discussed separately, in chapters 7 and 13, respectively.

## Current and Former Communist States

Physician complicity in torture has been pandemic in former and present Communist nations, defined to include the former Soviet Union, the Warsaw Pact nations of Eastern Europe, and the non-European nations of China, North Korea, and Cuba. Physicians in Communist nations (e.g., Albania,[3] Azerbaijan,[4] Belarus,[5] Bulgaria,[6] Kosovo,[7] Kyrgyzstan,[8] Macedonia,[9] Moldova,[10] Poland,[11] Romania,[12] Ukraine,[13] Uzbekistan,[14] and Tajikistan[15]) monitor torture, fail to record injuries, and write medical reports that do not record torture. As evidence, official false-negative medical records generally override differing findings by civilian physicians.[16] This anecdote comes from Kazakhstan, where a doctor ultimately registered minor bruises of unspecified cause on Mr. Polienko:

> After an extensive beating, the police pushed Mr. Polienko to the floor, put the plastic bag over his head and began to suffocate him. Then Mr. P. dragged Polienko to the middle of the room, ordered his colleague to sit on Polienko's legs, and started suffocating Polienko with the plastic bag from behind while pushing against Polienko's back with his knees. During the entire ordeal, Mr. Polienko remained handcuffed with his arms fixed behind the back. At the same time, an officer named Mr. M. kicked him in his side. . . .
>
> In the early morning of 22 November 2006, Mr. Romanov brought Mr. Polienko to the Schuchinsk Central District Hospital in order to receive a

medical-check-up necessary for his admittance to the preliminary detention center. Before the examination, Mr. Romanov further intimidated Mr.
Polienko, threatened him not to raise any complaints with the doctor, and
punched him on his head and chest. During the examination, which was not
confidential and took place in the presence of Romanov, the doctor, Mr. B.,
asked Mr. Polienko if he had been beaten. Mr. Polienko replied by asking
the doctor if he would be interested in the truth. Hearing this, Mr. Romanov
started pushing Mr. Polienko with his fist and said to the doctor: "Don't
you know, they all say they have been beaten?" Doctor B. then said to Mr.
Polienko, "OK, if you don't want to, you don't have to say anything to me.
That's your business after all."[17]

In Albania, hospital doctors observed beatings of patients: "When I decided
to go to Gjirokastra hospital, Argjir Çela and his brothers came in the hospital and
in front of all doctors and nurses started beating me. I was taken by them and the
auto ambulance sent me to the police commissariat where they continued beating
me very bad in three sessions."[18]

In Latvia, medical exams were "conducted in the presence of prison officers."
Prisoners were "seen by the doctor through the bars of the cell door or in the medical unit whilst being handcuffed behind the back (including during dental interventions), and consultations with the psychiatrist and psychologist often took place in
a special interview room with the prisoner being placed in a cage-like cubicle."[19]

Many Communist countries used a distinctive form of medical torture during the Cold War. As mentioned in a previous chapter, a spurious diagnosis of
sluggish schizophrenia was used to label dissidents' ideas of reform as delusions.
The delusional dissidents were then committed to psychiatric hospitals (prisons
without appeal), where drugs and other treatments were used to disorient them or
cause painful muscle spasms or even coma from brain-damaging hypoglycemia.
Robert van Voren reviews such practices in Bulgaria, China, Cuba, Czechoslovakia, Hungary, Romania, Russia, the Soviet Union, Turkmenistan, Uzbekistan, and
Yugoslavia.[20]

North Korea has a large system of hellish labor prisons. Many prison "doctors" are prisoners themselves or medically inclined laypeople.[21] Credible sources
report that the doctors directly abuse prisoners:

> While I was there, three women delivered babies on the cement floor without
> blankets. . . . It was horrible to watch the prison doctor kicking the pregnant
> women with his boots. When a baby was born, the doctor shouted, "Kill it
> quickly. How can a criminal expect to have a baby? Kill it."
>
> The women covered their faces with their hands and wept. Even though
> the deliveries were forced by injection, the babies were still alive when born.
> The prisoner-nurses, with trembling hands, squeezed the babies' necks to
> kill them.[22]

This story illustrates how one incident of torture has many dimensions of abuse: (a) the birth is forced by drugs in order to conform to the prison schedule; (b) the doctor kicks the prisoner; (c) the doctor degrades the woman as a criminal who does not merit the right to have a child; (d) the doctor orders coprisoners to kill the newborn child; (e) the baby is killed in front of the mother; (f) the doctor deprives the woman of the experience of breastfeeding; (g) the doctor's action takes her future with a child from her; (h) the partner with whom she became pregnant is kept from her; and (i) the official collusion among the prison, the doctor, and the other prisoner-attendants emphasizes the prisoner's powerlessness and hopelessness.

In the nations that emerged from the former Yugoslavia, doctors certify prisoners for harsh punishment, such as restraints or solitary confinement.[23] In Kosovo, for example, "one of the two prisoners was allegedly taken by members of the Special Unit to the Prison School and beaten there, whilst being held on the ground and handcuffed, in the presence of the Prison Director (as well as prisoners). Subsequently, the prisoner concerned was apparently taken to the disciplinary section (Block 5) and seen by a doctor, who declared him fit for punishment (which did not prevent the prisoner from being transferred to hospital, two days later)."[24]

## Western Europe

This geographic-political grouping includes all European nations (except Turkey) not included in the previous section. Four stand out for physician complicity and impunity for torture. (I exclude police brutality against immigrants and Romani.) Spain, Portugal, and Germany are discussed here, and as mentioned, the United Kingdom is discussed in chapter 7.

Medical complicity with brutal treatment of prisoners occurs in Spain.[25] State physicians do not disclose their names to prisoners and do not investigate or record the cause or severity of injuries that prisoners report to have been inflicted by police.[26] Physicians perform perfunctory exams of prisoners alleging torture, certify prisoners for brutal interrogations and isolation, and do not give prisoners their medical records to use in complaints about mistreatment.[27] Some Spanish doctors directly supervise the abuse of medically frail persons. This is a typical report from the Council of Europe:

> During the first medical examination he [the prisoner] said nothing. The doctor did not ask him any specific questions about his treatment by the Civil Guards but only asked whether he had anything to declare. The examination included auscultation [with a stethoscope] of the chest, blood pressure and pulse. After the examination, he was again blindfolded and stripped naked. At the second forensic medical examination, he told the doctor about his treatment by the Civil Guard because he was desperate and afraid. He told the doctor he had been subjected to "la bolsa" [a plastic bag over the head

to induce suffocation]. The doctor wrote down his complaints and said that he would inform the judge and try to visit him two to three times per day. He felt that his appearance must have been very poor at this time and with a marked deterioration from the first examination. At the second forensic medical examination the doctor became more serious when he observed his pulse. He overheard the doctor say that, "this was not the time or place to have an accident." The doctor saw that his head was a little bit red but there was no bruising.

After the second forensic medical examination the Civil Guards told him that they had been watching and that he should not have told anything to the doctor. However, the number of blows during the interrogation fell off thereafter and he was not again subjected to "la bolsa." He was also allowed to continue to wear his clothing and was not again interrogated naked.[28]

In Portugal, the security forces' physicians assist torture, fail to document injuries from torture, certify prisoners for prolonged restraint, and study prisoners' ability to withstand it.[29] Doctors have certified prisoners as fit for close confinement and perform cursory exams on prisoners who claim to be abused by prison staff.[30]

France tortured during the Algerian War of 1954–62 and also during the First Indochina War. There is some evidence of doctors abetting this torture.[31] The recent release of French archives should be a valuable resource for research.[32]

As noted, Germany protected its Nazi torture doctors. Nazi doctors easily concealed their brutal pasts during the postwar denazification, through which the Allies tried to prevent Nazis from obtaining senior positions in postwar Germany.[33] Although the government set up a modest program to identify, pursue, and prosecute Nazi criminals, the West German Medical Assembly did not censure or punish individual Nazi doctors.[34] Some Nazi doctors were recruited to US military research via Operation Paperclip (see chapter 5). Others associated with brutal crimes (e.g., Heinrich Berning, Hans Harmsen, Hans Reiter, Kurt Blome, and Julius Hallervorden) slipped quietly back into practice. Some, such as Dr. Hans Eppinger, who forced concentration camp prisoners to drink seawater, were highly honored for new medical work after the war.[35] Dr. Aribert Heim performed several hundred operations at the Mauthausen concentration camp, where he, often without anesthesia, injected prisoners' hearts with gasoline while recording the time it took the prisoners to die and the cost of the gasoline. After the war he quietly moved into private practice.[36] Dr. Werner Heyde, one of the few doctors caught by Nazi chasers, committed suicide in Germany just before his trial in 1959.[37] In 1964 Dr. Erich Fromm, a brown shirt and Schutzstaffel (SS) doctor, became the second president of the German Medical Association.[38] In response to a request that the association investigate and disqualify twenty-four doctors who allegedly oversaw the murder of about two hundred thousand persons with lethal injections, he presciently remarked, "I feel certain that the profession will be cleared following this investigation."[39]

In 1992 the WMA selected German physician Dr. Hans Joachim Sewering as its president-elect. During World War II Sewering had been in the SS, the Nazi organization most responsible for genocidal killings, when he sent more than nine hundred disabled children to be murdered. After the war Sewering held many prominent positions in German medicine, eventually rising to become president of the German Medical Association. Notwithstanding its position that Nazi doctors should be prosecuted and expelled from the profession (see chapter 5), the WMA defended Sewering against the international uproar over his nomination by noting his youth, the exigencies of war, coercion, his ignorance, and the lack of a criminal conviction.[40] Sewering was forced to forgo the WMA presidency. At the time he churlishly explained that he was forced to withdraw because of "severe damage [to the WMA] that could result from the Jewish World Congress."[41] In 2008, fifteen years after that debacle, Germany gave Sewering its highest medical honor.[42] His obituary did not mention his Nazi past.[43]

By 2012 the German medical community was again challenged by newly released archives showing the central role of Nazi physicians in promoting eugenics, euthanasia, genocide, and murderous "research." The medical association again declined to assert the personal accountability of medical collaborators with the Holocaust. It instead asserted a broad cultural responsibility for these crimes: "The crimes committed by Nazi medicine were not those of a few isolated and fanatical doctors, but rather took place with the substantial involvement of leading representatives of the medical association and medical specialisms as institutional bodies, as well as with the considerable participation of eminent representatives of university medicine and renowned biomedical research facilities."[44] The German Medical Association's concept of broad responsibility was, in effect, a general amnesty for individual Nazi physicians.

In 1990, after the reunification of East and West Germany, the German Medical Association did not seek to identify or hold accountable any physician who worked for East Germany's notorious Ministry for State Security (Stasi) in its torture prisons from 1950 to 1989.[45]

## Asia

Torture is widespread in the nations of Asia from the Middle East to the Pacific Ocean. Many regimes restrict human rights organizations' access to prisons, thereby making it difficult to determine the extent of medical complicity. The Human Rights Commission of Asia, Human Rights Watch, and Amnesty International maintain websites reporting physician complicity with torture in at least Bangladesh,[46] India,[47] Iran, Iraq,[48] Jordan,[49] Myanmar,[50] Nepal,[51] New Guinea,[52] Pakistan, the Philippines,[53] Sri Lanka,[54] Syria,[55] Thailand,[56] and Vietnam.[57] In Kuwait, officials have obstructed autopsies of persons or have falsified medical records or autopsy findings to conceal torture.[58] Three-fourths of a sample of India's 700,000 physicians have seen a tortured person. An astonishing one in seven have witnessed torture.[59] In the Republic of Turkey, some doctors assist torture despite the valiant resistance of the Turkish Medical Association and individual physicians. The Turkish government responded to the association's activism by creating a medical association for military and prison doctors that exempted them from civilian medical association oversight.[60]

The Republic of the Philippines is a member of the WMA. Human rights investigators have found evidence that its doctors collude with torture:

> [A student was arrested and beaten in a police detention center.] Three days later, a prison doctor examined him and signed a medical certificate stating that he bore no signs of ill-treatment even though he had signs of bruising on his stomach and head and had told the doctor of his treatment at the hands of the intelligence officer. After his release, the detainee filed a court complaint against the officer, but it was dismissed on the basis of the medical certificate.
>
> In another case, Vicente Ladlad, who was detained in 1983 and held in solitary confinement for two years and nine months, states that in his first week of solitary confinement guards never allowed him to sleep and threatened him with "salvaging" (extrajudicial execution by military or paramilitary agents) for failing to co-operate with his interrogators. On the sixth day, he ran a fever and was examined by a doctor. After the examination, Ladlad says, the doctor turned to his interrogator and said: "Kaya pa niya" ("He can still take it").[61]

Several reports examine the complicity of Israeli physicians with torture.[62] The Israel Medical Association is under international pressure for failing to address the underreporting of medical observations of torture-related injuries in prisons.[63]

## Africa

Torture occurred in all parts of Africa during and after post–World War II decolonization. This example from Algeria is typical:

> His body was stretched and . . . he was tortured with the chiffon method (a rag is pushed into the mouth and dirty water, urine or liquid chemicals are poured on it) and electric shocks. One of his torturers reportedly put his thumbs on Boubker Sadek's eyes and pressed, damaging his eyes. Apparently as a result of the trauma and injuries sustained under torture and ensuing lack of medical care during garde à vue [police] detention, Boubker Sadek lost the use of his left eye. Boubker Sadek reported that he received medical care only after he had been brought before the judicial authorities on 17 September 2002 and a medical examination was carried out upon his transfer to Serkadji prison in Algiers. Four days later he was admitted to the prison hospital where doctors apparently diagnosed detachment of the retina, a condition which may be facilitated by severe trauma and requires

prompt surgery. Between September 2002 and January 2003, he underwent two operations, but neither managed to rectify the damage to his eye. He says that his condition deteriorated during his imprisonment and that the sight in his other eye has weakened. Boubker Sadek says that he asked the doctor who treated him to issue a certificate about his medical condition, but the doctor reportedly refused, saying that he could not do so without permission from his superior.[64]

There are similar reports from Algeria,[65] Mauritania,[66] Morocco,[67] Namibia,[68] Senegal,[69] Swaziland,[70] Tunisia,[71] Yemen,[72] and Zambia.[73] Kenya's Prison Rule 24 requires medical officers to monitor prisoners during corporal punishment, and another law bars clinicians from saying that government policy conflicts with medical ethics.[74] Egypt's prison doctors participate in torture, cover up deaths by torture, and reportedly have operated on political prisoners without anesthesia.[75]

South Africa inflicted horrendous abuses against prisoners during its apartheid era. Dr. Wendy Orr noted that district medical surgeons were widely complicit with torture; she was transferred to other duties after she sued to prevent torture.[76] Physicians monitored "authorized" whippings.[77] In South Africa's Aversion Project, clinicians used electrical aversion therapy, an antiscientific "cure" for homosexuality.[78] The Medical Association of South Africa was a charter member of the WMA when that organization stated that doctors should be held personally accountable for crimes against humanity. Yet, after apartheid had fallen, the South African association apologized for the medical profession's collective failure without trying to address individual apartheid-era physicians' complicity with torture. The medical association tabled calls for a medical truth and reconciliation commission.[79] The long-delayed punishment of two physicians for complicity in the torture and murder of antiapartheid activist Dr. Stephen Biko is discussed in chapter 11.

## The Western Hemisphere

Anecdotes of medical torture in Latin America are hard to find because the prisons are difficult to survey. There are anecdotes about torture doctors in Bolivia,[80] Peru,[81] and Venezuela.[82] International human rights advocates have put together rich material from Mexico; this material is cited and described in chapter 4 and the appendix. The work of torture doctors in Argentina, Brazil, Chile, and Uruguay is discussed in relation to those countries' efforts to hold torture doctors accountable.

## Physician-Assisted Torture:
## Mutilation, Flogging, and Sexual Torture

I now shift from geography to consider three medically assisted techniques of torture: mutilation, flogging, and medico-sexual torture. Mutilation refers to cutting off or maiming the body so that the body is permanently damaged or disfigured. Amputation is one form of mutilation.

Amputations are performed by a dwindling number of Islamic authorities. This technique entails cutting off the right hand, both hands, fingers, or the right hand and left foot (cross amputation). Doctors have assisted with amputations in Libya, Mali, Sudan, Nigeria, and other countries.[83] Asian countries outside the Middle East, with the exception of Afghanistan, are not noted for recruiting doctors to assist in this practice.[84] A Libyan law of 1972 spells out the medical role in amputations as follows: (1) a medical examination must confirm that there is no illness or pregnancy and, if there is, propose a later date for the punishment; (2) the amputation may be performed at a hospital or at a prison clinic with anesthesia; (3) a period of clinical observation must follow the amputation to prevent complications.[85] A British-trained Sudanese surgeon trained guards to perform amputations:

> I devised the operation. I wanted the thing done quickly and without pain. I trained the guards in the prison where to give the local anesthetic and how to clean the hand. I trained them how to use the surgical scalpel. I wanted it to be done so that the patient [*sic*] would not lose blood. . . . I attended the first six or seven just to make sure my system was working all right, to see if there was anything to improve. I am very happy that it went without accident, not a single infection.[86]

In apparent deference to local cultural views, the WMA and the International Committee of the Red Cross (ICRC) have offered muted criticisms of punitive amputations. The ICRC published an incoherent written statement in a journal, saying it would "state its objection to amputations based on sharia but not do so publicly . . . [and it will] inform all health professionals of its position." It also said that Red Cross medical facilities and personnel may not be used for amputations.[87] The WMA did not respond to a 2005 article in *The British Medical Journal* calling for it to take a position on punitive amputations.[88] The BMA's convoluted position is discussed in chapter 7.

Oddly, the WMA's, ICRC's, and BMA's culturally deferential positions differ from Islamic-centered medical societies' forthright assertions that physicians should not be involved in punitive amputations. In Mauritania, after doctors had participated in several amputations, the national medical association successfully petitioned the government not to require doctors to participate, and since then the amputations have become less common.[89] The Nigerian Medical Association opposes doctor assistance with punitive amputations (although Nigerian physicians remain silent as police drop tortured bodies at mortuaries or on hospital grounds).[90] The Declaration of Kuwait, adopted by the International Conference of Islamic Medical Associations in 1981, asserts, "The physician shall not permit any of his special knowledge to be used to harm, destroy or inflict damage on the body, mind or spirit whatever the military or political issues. The physician's aim shall be to offer treatment and cure to the needy, be he friend or foe."[91] The Islamic Medical Association of North America (IMANA) opposes physician assistance with punitive amputations: "IMANA recommends that its members and all Muslim physicians as well as all physicians of conscience world wide do not participate in the delivery of inhumane treatment, lethal injection, non-surgical amputation or torture of inmates or political prisoners by any means when ordered by their employers, any government or private agencies or on their own. When asked to do so, not only should they refuse to comply but also notify human rights organizations such as Physicians for Human Rights."[92]

Amnesty International, the African Centre for Justice and Peace Studies (ACJPS), Human Rights Watch, REDRESS, and Physicians for Human Rights (PHR) all have called for punitive amputations to be deemed torture.[93] Amnesty International simply asserts, "This cruel and inhuman treatment, which is banned under international law, needs to be abolished immediately."[94]

There are other examples of medically assisted mutilation. In Iran in 2009, physicians assisted in blinding a man as a punishment for his blinding a child. Saudi Arabia inflicts blinding as well, although it is not clear if there is physician involvement.[95] During Kenya's war for independence from Great Britain, British soldiers spread-eagled prisoners in the prison yard and castrated them. The castrated prisoners were taken to the hospital, where doctors sewed up the wounds and returned the men to the cellblocks.[96] I cannot find any reports of physicians either protesting these injuries or being held accountable for complicity with them.[97] In 2013 Britain compensated the victims of these atrocities without apologizing.

Physician supervision of flogging appears to have spread from the United Kingdom throughout the Commonwealth to Afghanistan, Anguilla, Antigua, Australia,[98] Barbuda, the Bahamas, Barbados, Belize, Bermuda, Brunei,[99] Canada,[100] Egypt, the United Arab Emirates,[101] Grenada, Hong Kong,[102] India,[103] Indonesia, Iran,[104] Ireland, Jamaica, Jordan,[105] Kenya, Malaysia,[106] New Zealand, Nigeria, Pakistan, Qatar,[107] Saudi Arabia,[108] Sierra Leone, Singapore,[109] South Africa,[110] and Sri Lanka (see chapter 7). Nigeria flogs women for premarital sex if a doctor finds them healthy enough to be flogged.[111] Iran employs doctors to monitor flogging for various offenses, including those relating to sexual transgressions. Aceh province (Indonesia's only province allowed to have a sharia code of justice) flogs persons for religious transgressions, including homosexuality, under medical supervision.[112] The state of Victoria in Australia flogged its last prisoner in 1958, but there is no record of medical attention in that case.[113]

Pakistan's 1979 Execution of Punishment of Whipping Ordinance specifies that the whipping should be carried out in a public place in the presence of an authorized medical officer. The doctor is required to examine the prisoner before flogging "to ensure that the execution of the punishment will not cause the death of the convict." When flogging is delayed because of illness, a doctor must indicate when the prisoner becomes fit for the punishment.[114] In Kenya, although torture is constitutionally barred, Prison Rule 24(I) states,

> The medical officer shall examine a prisoner . . .
> (c) before the prisoner undergoes corporal punishment or any other punishment likely to affect his health, and shall certify whether the prisoner is fit to undergo the punishment;
> (d) during the course of infliction of corporal punishment.[115]

An Amnesty International report describes Malaysia's use of medically monitored whipping in detail. The whipping canes are soaked in saltwater to make them heavy and the lacerations painful. The cane is applied as hard as possible by muscular men who pull back at the end of the stroke to remove skin and fat. A doctor supervises each caning. "He checked my heart and blood pressure. He was a real doctor, didn't say a word. . . . He didn't reject anyone. Everyone was approved for whipping," said Mohd Jamil, a forty-nine-year-old Malaysian who was caned in 2006.[116] None of the victims reported being informed of the medical reason for the physician exam or being asked for medical information relevant to the punishment. Dr. Mohd Nisha was a young hospital physician who was asked to assist in a caning of two prisoners at Kajang Prison in 1996:

> "Witnessing it was part of my duty," she said. "Caning is quite painful to watch, no matter what. It's very traumatic to witness this." . . . Nevertheless, she emphasized that she was not forced to participate. "We have liberty to choose to go or not to go. They didn't pressurize me. But did they tell me about the terrible crime committed," Dr. Nisha explained. To persuade her to participate, prison officials told her that the two caning victims were responsible for raping a 13-year-old girl, right in front of the girl's parents. "I can't say it was the right thing," said Dr. Nisha, referring to the five or six strokes each prisoner received. "If you go to prison for 14 years, you're already punished." Afterwards, Dr. Nisha never participated in a caning session again.[117]

These anecdotes show that the doctor's role is to grant pro forma authorization to the flogging, that is, a superficial exam enables torture rather than restricts it. Sometimes a doctor might break the flogging into segments so that the entire sentence can be completed. Physicians also revive persons who lose consciousness during flogging so that they are conscious for the entire punishment. In all these roles the physicians are promoting the sentence rather than protecting the medical interests of the prisoner. Human rights groups have persuaded many Commonwealth countries to give up flogging; the notable exceptions are a dwindling number of Islamic nations, notably the Gulf States, Indonesia, Pakistan, Malaysia, and Singapore. Chapters of the Pakistan Medical Association oppose physician involvement in flogging.[118]

Afghanistan, Cameroon, Egypt, Kenya, Lebanon, Malawi, Romania, Tanzania, Tunisia, Turkmenistan, Uganda, the United Arab Emirates, and Zambia have medicalized sexual torture.[119] A Tunisian government forensic expert insists that anal exams on forcibly restrained prisoners were done with consent, but in all four cases detailed the "consent" was obtained by force, intimidation, and beatings.[120] In Lebanon, as in Egypt, forcible medical rectal exams are carried out on gay men despite protests and promises to stop the practice.[121] In some of these countries, a brutal medical rectal exam or sodomy with a baton is performed on the false pretense that it can assess for homosexuality. In others, including Afghanistan, vaginal examinations are forcibly performed with the incorrect rationalization that they can assess the virginity or sexual orientation of women who are suspected of violating sexual mores or secular or religious laws.[122] Ironically, Egypt protects doctors who perform virginity exams on prisoners even though it has penalties for doctors who perform female genital mutilation.[123] An Egyptian military doctor who performed virginity exams on women prisoners in exam rooms while guards watched from the hall was recently cleared of "criminal indecency."[124] In 2017 the WMA came out against anal examinations to assess homosexuality, although this resolution is oddly silent on the equally spurious and abusive virginity exam performed on women prisoners.[125]

A map of torture doctors entirely overlaps the global map of torture. It includes fascist autocracies and democratic republics, rich countries and poor ones. It is therefore reasonable to estimate that torture doctors ply their trade in more than a hundred countries. Although estimating how many physicians abet torture is not possible, it is clear that every torturing nation can find enough doctors to carry out its torture policies.

# 7

# THE PARADOX OF
# THE UNITED KINGDOM

The United Kingdom merits an expanded consideration in this book for several reasons. First, in July 1945, two months before World War II ended, the BMA hosted the organizing committee for what would become the WMA in London. Second, British authors largely drafted the WMA's 1948 Declaration of Geneva (originally the Charter of Medicine), asserting physicians' duty to comply with international law. The BMA and the American Medical Association (AMA) have played and continue to play leadership roles in WMA funding and policymaking. Third, Amnesty International was founded in the United Kingdom and has taken a leadership role in addressing medical complicity with torture. Finally, the United Kingdom has a troubled history of its own physicians abetting torture, especially regarding the practice of medically supervised flogging and during the Troubles in Northern Ireland. Despite being at the center of efforts to condemn torture doctors, the United Kingdom and the BMA have been reticent on the matter of holding torture doctors accountable.

This chapter begins in 1949, after the BMA's formative work in creating the WMA. That year the BMA submitted the report "War Crimes and Medicine" to the WMA's third assembly in Geneva.[1] The BMA bluntly recommended "judicial action by which members of the medical profession who shared in war crimes are punished." The WMA accepted the BMA recommendation for "judicial punishment" of physicians and said that it would expel "members who have been personally guilty of the crimes."[2] This was an odd statement in that the "members" of the WMA are national medical associations rather than individual physicians.

In 1961 a British lawyer, Peter Benenson, founded the Appeal for Amnesty (now called Amnesty International) after learning of two Portuguese students who were imprisoned for toasting "freedom" in a bar. Benenson's op-ed about the students struck a nerve in the British public.[3] Amnesty International organized letter-writing campaigns to government leaders on behalf of "prisoners of conscience" who had been imprisoned for expressing opinions dissenting from their governments. Later Amnesty International campaigns expanded to advocate for any prisoner at risk of medical neglect, torture, or capital punishment.

A scandal compelled Amnesty to focus on medicalized torture by its home country. In 1971 the public became aware that the British government was torturing prisoners in Northern Ireland and that physicians and psychologists monitored the torture and misled investigators about the aftereffects. In November the government appointed the Lord Chief Justice of England, Lord Parker of Waddington, to investigate the matter. The Parker report concluded that the interrogation techniques being used were illegal.[4] Ireland sued Britain in the European Commission of Human Rights, which in 1976 ruled that Britain had tortured.[5] Then the European Court of Human Rights took up the matter. Although that court never saw United Kingdom memos explicitly authorizing torture, it found that the techniques used on prisoners from Northern Ireland were "inhuman and degrading treatment" and "torture."[6]

In December 1972, a few months after the Parker report was issued, Amnesty International launched its Campaign for the Abolition of Torture. Amnesty cited the Parker report and torture reports from six other countries.[7] The campaign's budget of USD 62,000 came from small donations.[8] Britain's premier medical journals, the BMA's *British Medical Journal* and *The Lancet*, editorialized in favor of medical association codes condemning physician complicity with torture.[9] Amnesty International hosted conferences, issued damning country reports, and won a Nobel Peace Prize. In 1973 Amnesty proposed a medical ethics code that included methods for investigating doctors who had allegedly tortured.[10] The United Nations defined torture in 1975.[11] That same year the WMA passed its momentous Declaration of Tokyo, which banned physician collaboration with torture (see chapter 10).

Nine years later, in 1984, the BMA convened a working party to investigate the claim "that some doctors appear to be cooperating in torture" in Northern Ireland.[12] In 1986 the working party found "incontrovertible evidence of doctors' involvement in planning and assisting in torture, not only under duress, but also voluntarily." Although the working party was convened because of concerns about Great Britain's clinicians' collaboration with torture in Northern Ireland, it skimmed over evidence of torture close to home by citing a softball British investigation without mentioning the harsh judgments of the European Commission of Human Rights or the ruling of the European Court of Human Rights. The working party instead focused on doctors assisting torture in the Soviet Union, Iraq, Uruguay, Romania, Brazil, and Chile and ignored widely known physician complicity with torture in Commonwealth nations such as India, Kenya, Malaysia, Mauritius, Nigeria, Pakistan, Uganda, and Yemen. It demurred to deceptive denials of torture from South Africa, Israel, and Tanzania. The geopolitically biased report also steered clear of cultural sensitivities. For example, it did not say that a doctor who assisted an amputation under an Islamic court's order was abetting torture.

The BMA's enthusiasm for holding torture doctors accountable steadily waned. In 1947, as noted previously, it had called for judicial punishment. In 1992 it recommended that doctors alleged to abet torture should be "fully and fairly investigated and that those found culpable are barred from medical practice and from membership in professional associations."[13] In 2001 the BMA wrote, "All organizations with an interest in human rights issues should be involved in campaigns for the prosecution of perpetrators of serious human rights violations, including health professionals who are complicit with and advise torturers. In effect, this means opposing impunity measures wherever they exist. . . . The WMA has resolved that national medical bodies should prevent doctors who have committed abuses from evading justice."[14] This was an odd statement given that by 2001, as discussed in chapter 5, the WMA had long abandoned any pretense of interest in holding torture doctors accountable. In 2009 the BMA said that it would not investigate cases of individual physicians.[15]

Even aside from the late twentieth-century Troubles in Northern Ireland, the United Kingdom and the BMA had reason to be reticent about holding torture doctors accountable. British colonies' struggles for independence after World War II were bloody affairs. From the 1950s to the 1970s, British forces brutally suppressed independence movements in the British Cameroons, Brunei, British Guiana, Borneo/Malaysia, Cyprus, Kenya, and Yemen (Aden). There are many reports of torture in Yemen, where the British refused to let Red Cross inspectors into its prisons or to allow prisoners' access to their own doctors.[16] Castration in Kenya was discussed in chapter 6. Contrary to its strong endorsement of medical truth commissions in 1986—"to establish the truth and allow victims to have a hearing"—the BMA has not convened a truth commission to excavate the history of UK physicians' collaboration with torture.[17] Recently opened archives of the Colonial Administration should illuminate these sordid histories.[18]

In 2014 two credible human rights groups detailed a total of fifty-eight allegations of UK doctors' involvement in the torture of Iraqi prisoners between 2003 and 2008.[19] For example,

[At the Al Shaibah Detention Centre] the male doctor who visited me was a Captain. The interpreter introduced him to me. The Captain insisted that I take my clothes off but I refused. It is against my religion to be naked in front of strangers. I refused and [Sergeant] Swede came in with around 3 to 4 soldiers who were all holding batons. He told me that if I didn't take my clothes off, they would beat me with the batons. I knew they would do this, as they had been doing it since my arrest. I felt extremely threatened. I felt obliged to do it and I took my clothes off. The doctor was standing nearby watching this happen. I thought he looked quite young. He asked me to lie on a stretcher naked. He carried out a very quick check on me and asked me whether I was suffering from any conditions. I told the doctor about the beatings I had suffered since my arrest and the injury to my stomach from the hammer. I told him how much pain I was in because of this. He told me he thought I had a stomach ulcer. He said this without examining me, or looking in my throat or taking an x-ray of my stomach. He listened to what I said about the pain and the beatings and made no comment except to diagnose an ulcer. I told him that I had never had anything wrong with my stomach before, until the soldier had smashed me in it with the hammer. The doctor told me he would write me a prescription for an orange tablet that would help but he did not say what this was. My t-shirt and shorts were covered in blood from the beating to my face and in particular my nose. The doctor could clearly see this and didn't ask me about it. I told him about the injury I had received to my nose and that I thought it was broken because it was so swollen but he didn't do or say anything.

The 2003 death of Baha Mousa, a British prisoner in Basra, Iraq, was the exception to physician impunity. Mousa was apparently innocent of any crime. He was picked up (for reasons unknown) and taken to a prison under United Kingdom control. One evening, Mousa, whose head was covered with a bag, was assaulted by a group of soldiers who beat him and kicked him. He died of asphyxia with multiple signs of severe trauma. Several courts eventually ruled on the case.[20] A soldier-physician, Dr. Derek Keilloh, had unsuccessfully attempted to resuscitate Mousa. He did not report that the body was battered. In 2012 Keilloh's license was revoked for ignoring the needs of a torture victim, failing to report the abuse, and lying to investigators.[21] The penalty against Keilloh appears to be unique in the long history of British medical complicity with torture.

Other anecdotes bear mentioning. The United Kingdom briefly suspended the license of an immigrant Iraqi doctor, Mohammed Kassim Al-Byati, who saw and treated tortured prisoners in one of Saddam Hussein's prisons (see chapter 2).[22] Britain continues to allow Vincent Bajinya, a Rwandan doctor charged with genocide, to practice.[23] This is despite the BMA's endorsement of a WMA code stating, "A physician who perpetrates [torture, war crimes, or crimes against humanity] . . . is unfit to practice medicine."[24]

## Flogging

Physician-supervised flogging (also known as whipping or caning) is unusual in international torture in that the United Kingdom seems to have exported this practice throughout its colonies, protectorates, and Commonwealth members. Here I exclude a common form of torture called falanga or bastinado in which the soles of the feet are caned or whipped; medical oversight of this technique is not described. Medically supervised flogging is described in chapter 6. Although Great Britain banned most flogging in 1948, it continued to impose medically supervised flogging up to the 1970s for a few offenses committed inside prisons as well for crimes in its former colonies and against separatists in Northern Ireland.[25] As late as the mid-1960s, a British physician could clear a prisoner for flogging before the prisoner was tied to a frame and whipped with a birch rod or cat o' nine tails (named for its nine whips, which left scars like the claw of a cat).[26] In 2001, twenty-six years after it had endorsed the WMA Declaration of Tokyo, the BMA finally spoke against physician collaboration in penal amputations or flogging without asserting that physicians supervising such punishments were abetting torture.[27] In opposing flogging as a matter of policy without defining it as torture, the BMA sidestepped the issue of whether medical boards should hold doctors who oversaw floggings accountable for abetting torture.

Although the prevalence of medically abetted flogging is decreasing, the leading countries where flogging is practiced are mostly members of the former British Empire. Therefore, it is fair to propose that the United Kingdom bears a special responsibility for working to end this abuse. Toward that end the BMA should

- assert that flogging is torture;
- assert that a physician who clears a person for flogging, monitors flogging, treats or certifies a prisoner for continued flogging after it begins, or fails to report each case of flogging to human rights groups is committing a breach of medical professionalism and abetting torture;
- assert that any physician or nurse who abets flogging should be subject to licensing sanctions and the case data should be referred to a criminal prosecutor;
- apologize for Britain's role in creating and disseminating legal codes and models for the practice of medically monitored flogging;
- compensate victims of flogging within the United Kingdom, including those from Northern Ireland or any other location where a person was flogged under Britain's auspices (n.b., the Convention Against Torture says "each State Party shall ensure in its legal system that the victim of an act of torture obtains redress and has an enforceable right to fair and adequate compensation, including the means for as full rehabilitation as possible");[28]
- compile and publish periodic reports assessing the progress of each formerly UK-affiliated country in meeting the above standards; and
- lobby to have the WMA adopt analogous policy for this widespread form of medically abetted torture.

The United Kingdom's medical community led the world in highlighting the problem of physician complicity with torture. One can only speculate whether national pride or shame over its long history of medically abetted torture has blunted the BMA's pursuit of its own torture doctors and its commitment to abolish the practice of medically abetted flogging. The loss of that kind of leadership is a loss for the global community.

# PART III

## HUMANISTS AND HEALERS

# 8

# HUMANISTS FOR HUMAN RIGHTS

A global human rights movement emerged from the horrors of World War II. It was new in the way it broadened the Enlightenment agenda for democratic republics, universal suffrage, religious tolerance, and the abolition of slavery to include diverse human rights and eventually new forms of justice, such as compensation and accountability for injustice. It built new institutions, including the United Nations. The institutions, in turn, adopted new international laws, such as the Convention on the Prevention and Punishment of the Crime of Genocide in 1948 and the Geneva Conventions to protect noncombatants in times of war. And then countless humanists and advocates created new nongovernmental human rights organizations, such as Amnesty International and Human Rights Watch. Eventually, this movement turned its attention to the impunity of torture doctors.

Franklin and Eleanor Roosevelt may be fairly credited with articulating the modern right not to be tortured. In trying to mobilize Americans to confront the menace of Nazism, President Roosevelt gave his "Four Freedoms" speech to Congress in 1941, shortly before the attack on Pearl Harbor. In that address he asserted that all people were entitled to four freedoms: freedom of speech, freedom of religion, freedom from want, and freedom from fear. After the war President Harry Truman delegated to Eleanor the task of continuing the human rights effort, which led to her chairing the Commission of Human Rights to draft a bill of rights for the UN.[1] She sought views beyond the politically calibrated positions of national delegates, soliciting aspirational rights from voices in civil society, such as church leaders, labor leaders, and intellectuals. She engaged articulate philosophers and humanists, such as India's Mahatma Gandhi, Aldous Huxley (author of *Brave New World*), and others. She believed that ordinary citizens and civil society would create a "curious grapevine" to carry human rights into the affairs of nations.[2] She insisted that the document that would become the

Universal Declaration of Human Rights be more than a general homage to the concept of human rights but that it enumerate specific rights. The declaration's preamble shows how it posited respect for human rights as central to the effort to prevent war and build peace:

> Whereas recognition of the inherent dignity and of the equal and inalienable rights of all members of the human family is the foundation of freedom, justice and peace in the world,
>     Whereas disregard and contempt for human rights have resulted in barbarous acts which have outraged the conscience of mankind.[3]

Article 5 of the declaration's thirty articles addresses torture: "No one shall be subjected to torture or to cruel, inhuman or degrading treatment or punishment."

The Universal Declaration of Human Rights became the template for decades of developing international human rights laws. The Geneva Conventions (1949); the European Convention on Human Rights (1950); the Covenant on Civil and Political Rights (1966); the International Covenant on Civil and Political Rights (1977); the Convention against Torture and Other Cruel, Inhuman or Degrading Treatment or Punishment (1984); and the Rome Statute of the International Criminal Court (1998) all cite article 5.

Eleanor Roosevelt's vision of a "curious grapevine" eventually became the human rights movement. Nongovernmental organizations, including labor unions, churches, student organizations, and journalists, mobilized public opinion to challenge governments to allow the realization of the declaration's enumerated rights.[4] Specialized human rights organizations, such as Amnesty International (1961), Human Rights Watch (1978), and Physicians for Human Rights (1981), emerged later.

It was fitting that Ms. Roosevelt added nongovernmental humanists to the voices of government officials in creating the Universal Declaration of Human Rights. Human rights protect the people and organizations of civil society. Governments' violations of human rights are often aimed at suppressing civil society by censoring the press, obstructing the organization of political parties, or engaging in torture. Torture is as often a weapon against a country's own citizens as it is a weapon of war against foreign enemies. Totalitarian regimes rejected the declaration's assertion of human rights as intruding on national sovereignty. An official Soviet newspaper, *Isvestia*, mocked Eleanor's "curious grapevine" as "weeds in the field." It said that human rights lobbyists at the UN were "rubbish that should be thrown out."[5] Despite decades of vicious reprisals by countless authoritarian leaders, the human rights movement has gained adherents.

In the mid-1970s the human rights movement turned a corner. Up to that time it had promoted human rights and advocated to protect persons who were endangered. Now, it shifted to confronting the impunity that protected government officials who violated human rights. It sought to identify, denounce, and secure the punishment of those officials. Although trials by the World Court or international tribunals could hold officials responsible for crimes against humanity, those trials were expensive, logistically difficult, politically charged, and usually aimed at senior government officials.[6] Human rights advocates addressed this problem by creating strategies for using domestic criminal and civil courts and other institutions of civil society against lower level government officials.[7] This shift set the stage for holding torture doctors accountable.

In the mid-1970s Portugal and Greece showed how domestic courts could act against dictators and torturers. On April 24, 1974, Portugal's military government collapsed during the Carnation Revolution. Portuguese courts subsequently tried hundreds of members of the International Police for the Defense of the State and General Directorate of Security for human rights abuses. On July 24 the collapse of the Regime of the Colonels in Greece led to similar trials. Greece, Hippocrates' homeland, inadvertently became the first country to punish a torture doctor.

Dr. Dimitrios Kofas was a low-ranking officer and physician with Greece's military police during a brutal junta that ruled from 1967 until 1974. He was one of hundreds of officials who were prosecuted for torture and other crimes after the junta fell. Kofas made rounds on prisoners who were being tortured. Some prisoners called him the "traffic controller" because he medically assessed prisoners undergoing torture and advised the guards when it was safe to continue or when the torture should be eased so that the prisoner did not die. He promised medications to ill prisoners and then failed to bring them. He promised drugs to a man with heart disease and four days later gave him four aspirin tablets. He offered orange juice to a man whose urine had turned orange from being kicked or beaten on his kidney. He dispensed orange juice so frequently to tortured prisoners that some prisoners called him the "orange juice doctor." He told the wife of a prisoner that he had sent her previously healthy husband to a military hospital with a stroke. At the hospital she found her husband with deep gashes on his legs, bruises on his shoulder, and his genitals black from trauma. Kofas was court-martialed on eleven charges of dereliction of duty and sentenced to seven years in prison but was soon released.[8] As far as I can determine, he has resumed practice in Greece.

On the surface the Kofas conviction seemed to change nothing. Organized medicine remained aloof from the human rights movement. It did not see Kofas's court-martial as a call for change or a sign of things to come. As far as I can determine, a decade passed before a medical human rights document stressed that Kofas was a physician.[9] Even so, the events in Portugal and Greece signaled a new age in human rights, and Kofas went down just like the other torturers in those trials. Accountability for torture doctors was under way.

## Literature and Torture Doctors

Lynn Hunt and Steven Pinker are among scholars who partly attribute the post-Enlightenment emergence of human rights to rising public exposure to novels.[10]

In this debated point of view, the association between reading great fiction and empathy is more than an association; novels appear to foster empathy between a reader and people in circumstances that the reader will never encounter.[11] In the latter half of the twentieth century, fiction advanced the public's understanding of torture as a political issue and a cause of enormous suffering. Some works belong both to the humanities and to the human rights movement. I exclude from this category nonfiction works such as Seiichi Morimura's *The Devil's Gluttony* (1980), which sold 2.5 million copies and provoked an extraordinary discussion in Japan of its medical torture during World War II. I also exclude nonfiction documentaries, such as *Doctors of the Dark Side*, a film about medical interrogators in war on terror prisons.[12] Some literary works about torture do not discuss doctors: for example, Margaret Atwood's poem "Footnote to the Amnesty Report on Torture," *The Colonel* by Carolyn Forché, or *One for the Road* by Harold Pinter.[13] In *Waiting for the Barbarians*, South African author J. M. Coetzee's magistrate defines the doctrine of interrogational torture this way: "Pain is truth; all else is subject to doubt."[14]

The first novel about a demonic doctor might be Mary Shelley's *Frankenstein* (1818).[15] It is not clear whether Jekyll was a physician or a scientist in Robert Louis Stevenson's *The Strange Case of Dr. Jekyll and Mr. Hyde* (1886).[16] A decade later H. G. Wells wrote *The Island of Dr. Moreau* (1896) about a sadistic medical scientist.[17] *The Cabinet of Dr. Caligari*, a 1920 German expressionist horror film, told the story of an asylum director who was a serial killer.[18] *The Great God Pan* (1894) and its 2013 feminist spinoff *Helen's Story* (2013) are two other mad-medical scientist novels.[19] None of these physicians or medical scientists are torture doctors in the sense of committing torture for governments. They are serial killers or megalomaniac psychopaths who inflict murder and pain and are driven by personal demons rather than government orders.

Fictional literature about torture doctors tends to explore their social, political, and institutional milieu rather than their psychopathologies. To what degree do orders, fear, loyalty, or political banality explain the torture doctor? What is the moral responsibility of a torture doctor for government crimes or for complicity with the government during a fascist political era? Does punishing a torturer atone for the crime? Can it?

Novels and dramas about Nazi doctors are the starting point of this genre. *Suspicion* (1952) was a pathbreaking, influential work telling of a concentration camp surgeon who changed his name and became the manager an elite clinic in Zurich after the war.[20] A Nazi-chasing detective gets himself admitted to the clinic. When the staff realize that he is pursuing the head physician, they try to kill the patient. This novel's publication in a popular magazine offered a German-speaking audience a provocative view of Nazi doctors' postwar careers. *Free Fall* (1959) tells of a Gestapo psychiatrist's interrogation of a British military POW.[21] *The Boys from Brazil* (1976) was a science fiction confection in which Auschwitz doctor Josef Mengele escaped to South America and began creating clones of Hitler to resurrect the Thousand-Year Reich.[22] *The Debt* (2011) is a film based on an Israeli novel about three Mossad agents who are sent to East Berlin to capture the infamous Nazi "Surgeon of Birkenau" and bring him to justice.[23] *The Chosen Ones: A Novel* (2016) is a fictionalization of the Nazi program of euthanizing disabled children.[24] Haruki Murakami's *Hard-Boiled Wonderland* (1993) is a deeply metaphorical analysis of the Holocaust and a medical scientist like Josef Mengele.[25]

The literature on Japanese torture doctors during World War II is smaller than that examining Nazi medicine. But both fiction and nonfiction accounts have resonated in Japan, where their history of torture medicine is less well known. Shusako Endo's *The Sea and Poison* (1986) tells of Dr. Suguro and his colleagues, who performed lethal experiments on prisoners during World War II. The book carefully explores questions of conscience, duty, medical professionalism, and finally, accountability:

> "Still, some day, we are going to have to answer for it," said Suguro, leaning close suddenly and whispering. "That's for sure. It's certain that we're going to have to answer for it."
>
> "Answer for it? To society? If it's only to society, it's nothing to get worked up about. . . . If those who are going to judge us had been put in the same situation, would they have done anything different? So much for the punishments of society."[26]

*Philosophy of a Knife* (2008) is a slasher movie that mixes real and studio footage to depict Japan's Nazi-like medical experiments at Unit 731.[27] Overall the books about World War II's torture doctors are a diverse lot. Some plumb the moral and psychological depths of torture medicine. Others have used World War II as a trope for one-dimensional allegories or cheap porn.

Two classic novels, *1984* and *A Clockwork Orange*, set the stage for the postwar discussion of torture doctors. They are both predicated on the fantasy that future governments might try to use torture to create ideal citizens (rather than to interrogate or punish). They also profoundly explore what people find most repellent about torture doctors, that is, the misuse of science and the abuse of humans.

George Orwell's *1984* (1949) describes a torturer, O'Brien, who works for the Ministry of Love in Big Brother's totalitarian dystopia. O'Brien and his white-coated assistants torture Winston to eliminate his capacity for love. O'Brien is a prescient depiction of the clinicians who worked for Soviet psychiatry and US interrogational behavioral science consultation teams. He has the skills of a psychologist, psychiatrist, and medical doctor:

> It was O'Brien who was directing everything. It was he who set the guards onto Winston and who prevented them from killing him. It was he who decided when Winston should scream with pain, when he should have a respite, when he should be fed, when he should sleep, when the drugs should be pumped into his arm. It was he who asked the questions and suggested the

answers. He was the tormentor, he was the protector, he was the inquisitor, he was the friend. And once—Winston could not remember whether it was in drugged sleep, or in normal sleep, or even in a moment of wakefulness—a voice murmured in his ear: "Don't worry, Winston; you are in my keeping. For seven years I have watched over you. Now the turning point has come. I shall save you, I shall make you perfect."[28]

*A Clockwork Orange* (1962) recounts how Dr. Branom and Dr. Brodsky torture Alex with aversion therapy. Like the characters in *1984*, they work with white-coated assistants in a high-tech clinic. They mock how they inadvertently destroy Alex's love of Beethoven, thereby showing that his behavior, not his humanity, is their only concern. The prison chaplain tells Alex,

> Very hard ethical questions are involved. You are to be made into a good boy number 6655321. Never again will you have the desire to offend in any way whatsoever against the State's Peace. . . . It may not be nice to be good, little 6655321. It may be horrible to be good. . . . You are passing now to a region beyond the reach of the power of prayer. A terrible thing to consider. And yet, in a sense, in choosing to be deprived of the ability to make an ethical choice, you have chosen to be good.[29]

Dr. Branom in turn tells Alex, "You are being made sane. You are being made healthy."[30]

In *1984* and *A Clockwork Orange*, medicalized torture is used to break and remake a prisoner into the state's ideal citizen. Winston is crushed into idolatry of Big Brother's invincible dictatorship. *A Clockwork Orange* has a surprisingly optimistic ending. The totalitarian regime employing the doctors in *A Clockwork Orange* somehow collapses. Out of prison and living in a nonfascist state, Alex rediscovers music and lives a normal life.

A third novel offers a false and menacing omen of the power of torture. *The Manchurian Candidate* (1959) tells how Dr. Yen Lo uses hypnosis to program an American prisoner during the Korean War to be a sleeper agent. The repatriated prisoner is activated and directed to assassinate a US presidential candidate.[31]

Writers announced the Soviet Union's use of psychiatric hospitals to torture political dissidents well before Western psychiatrists crusaded against the abuses. Valeriy Tarsis's novel *Ward 7* (1965) had an enormous impact in the Soviet Union and Europe (see chapter 11).[32] Tarsis, a dissident, drew on his experience of having been a prisoner-patient in Moscow's Kashchenko Hospital. His book creates *Ward 7* from Chekov's classic *Ward 6* (1893), which told the story of a tsarist insane asylum. The brutality of the neglectful nineteenth-century asylum was escalated by the intentional abuse in *Ward 7*. "Gorbunov and Gorchakov" (1970) is a poem by another former Soviet psychiatric prisoner describing a conversation between two prisoners in a Soviet psychiatric hospital between their interrogations by psychiatrists.[33] The play *Every Good Boy Deserves Favor* (1977) illuminates how the Soviet government was abusing dissidents with false psychotherapy.[34] By that time, however, the battle between Western and Soviet psychiatric professional organizations was well under way. Aleksandr Solzhenitsyn's *A Day in the Life of Ivan Denisovitch* (1962) and *Gulag Archipelago* mention the role of torture doctors in Stalin's camps.[35]

*Z* (1969) is an enormously influential novel about the Greek junta of Kofas.[36] An honest autopsy discovers that a dissident political leader was murdered, rather than killed by an accident, thereby highlighting the need for doctors to hold regimes accountable for crimes.

*Death and the Maiden* (1990) tells of a former prisoner in South America suffering from PTSD. During her imprisonment she had been blindfolded and repeatedly raped by a sadistic doctor. The novel explores the difficulties of traumatized persons' memory and an encounter with a man who might be her torturer.[37] Ariel Dorfman, the Chilean author, wrote this work as his country was coming to terms with the legacy of torture of Gen. Augusto Pinochet's military junta.[38]

*Anil's Ghost* (2000) tells of Dr. Anil Tissera, a forensic human rights pathologist who is trying to identify a murder victim in Sri Lanka to bring the responsible official to justice.[39] Michael Ondaatje, a Sri Lankan, wrote and released the book during the Sri Lankan Civil War.

Two major films depict the war on terror. A lavish Turkish movie, *Valley of the Wolves: Iraq* (2006) depicts events similar to the torture at Abu Ghraib. Its story of an American doctor who takes kidneys from wounded Iraqis and sends them to the United States to be transplanted into rich people illustrates the blowback of American medical torture.[40] The US film *Zero Dark Thirty* (2012) has a fiction of omission: it does not show the medical collaboration in torture.[41]

*The Little Red Chairs* (2016) imagines Dr. Vlad, a character like Serbia's notorious Dr. Radovan Karadžić, arriving as a mysterious fugitive in a small Irish village, where he introduces a destabilizing evil.[42] The title comes from a work of public art in which 11,541 red chairs (of which 643 were child size) were placed in the streets Sarajevo to memorialize the victims of the siege from 1992 to 1996.[43]

Witness literature is a genre in which survivors' stories preserve history and point to the need for accountability. In 2001 the Nobel Prize Committee devoted its centennial year to witness literature.[44] Holocaust witness literature is the best-known example of this genre and safeguards the truth of torture against revisionist deniers while demanding accountability by fostering empathy with the suffering of the survivors and victims. Two of Mengele's subjects wrote the notable example *Children of the Flames: Dr. Josef Mengele and the Untold Story of the Twins of Auschwitz*.[45] Jacobo Timerman's *Prisoner without a Name, Cell without a Number* (excerpt in chapter 2) is a memoir of being tortured in an Argentine prison.[46]

The most recent incarnation of the witness genre appears on social media. Blogs, tweets, and cell phone pictures and videos carry images and messages from and within societies burdened by torture. Images from both traditional journalists and laypeople quickly and broadly migrate through global social media networks. As in the pre–social media age, some images of torture can have a powerful effect on public opinion.[47] In Egypt, Tunisia, Pakistan, and Russia, cell phone images of torture posted on social media have led to the prosecution of guards.[48] The infamous photographs of torture at Abu Ghraib, which included smiling selfies of guards, spread widely on social media. Academic papers are only beginning to examine the effects of social media in documenting human rights abuses and in coordinating protests.[49] Elaborate "Denounces" against torture doctors and other regime officials are highly developed social media campaigns (see chapter 11).

By the mid-1970s the public considered torture a common violation of human rights in need of preventive intervention. That awareness set the stage for accountability. At this point torture abolitionists had to mobilize the medical community to improve forensic methods for trials. That task is where this book now turns.

# 9

# HEALERS FOR
# HUMAN RIGHTS

In the mid-1970s the human rights movement had few ties to the medical community. Churches, lay advocates for human rights, and lawyers were its core. To introduce evidence to bring torturers (including doctors) to justice, the movement needed medical experts who were willing and qualified to testify that a person had been tortured. That forensic testimony had to be based on sound science so that it could withstand withering cross-examinations. Ideally, the medical forensic skills had to be able to identify at least some forms of torture distinct from the kinds of trauma that might occur by accident or during ordinary criminal assault. The forensic medical science of torture also had to address the fact that torturing nations that were sensitive to international pressure were instructing officials to use "stealth torture," methods that did not leave readily apparent scars or other physical signs that could be detected by routine physical examinations or autopsies.[1] Torture-focused protocols for conducting autopsies and physical exams were needed to disprove governments' false autopsy reports, death certificates, and medical records. The questions were knotty. For example, was it possible to prove that a small scar under the skin where a former prisoner reported having been electrically shocked resulted from torture as opposed to an old spider bite? A forensic method was also needed to excavate mass graves of jumbled bodies that had often been burned with lime or gasoline bonfires in order to identify the individuals, detect torture, and tie, by timing and ballistic evidence, those deaths to the movements and weapons used by police and military units. Medical experts had to develop the skill to read death certificates (that were normally accepted as honest even if occasionally mistaken) to critically assess what was written and what was omitted and to illuminate implausible entries. The list was endless.

Few physicians were interested in such matters. Medical schools neither researched nor taught these topics. Medical associations were not inclined to go beyond condemning torture to develop protocols for evaluating torture-related injuries as they had for natural diseases, such as heart disease. Appeals by visionaries, such as Dr. Jonathan Mann, for the medical profession to embrace human rights as a means to improve public health were marginalized as idealistic, politically contentious, and tangential to the core clinical mission of medicine.[2] It is no surprise that Korey's encyclopedic history of the relationship between nongovernmental organizations and human rights devotes only a few vague pages to "The 'Unexplored Continent' of Physician Involvement in Human Rights."[3]

By 1973 Amnesty International was using "Urgent Action Appeals" to exhort its members to write to senior government officials on behalf of individual prisoners asking that the prisoner not be abused and that proper medical care and legal representation be made available.[4] Amnesty created the Health Professionals Network, which at its peak had ten thousand health professionals writing on behalf of hundreds of imprisoned clinicians and prisoners with serious health problems.[5] The network's volunteers and staff conducted educational programs on physician participation in torture. Amnesty was clear about its position that torture doctors should be held accountable: "The role of health professionals in abuses or in their cover-up should be investigated and those found guilty of illegal actions should be prosecuted."[6]

Centers for rehabilitation drew clinicians and led to a science for diagnosing and treating torture survivors. These centers arose from Amnesty International's campaigns against torture that began in 1972.[7] Amnesty, working with Danish, Chilean, Swedish, and Greek physicians, outlined the complex medical, legal, and social services needs of torture survivors from Gen. Augusto Pinochet's fascist rule in Chile. The centers drew their energy from the community of torture survivors and the human rights movement rather than from the mainstream medical or legal community. Torture survivors often assumed positions as clinicians, advocates, and charismatic leaders of the centers.[8] For example, Dr. José Quiroga cofounded the Program for Torture Victims, the first such program in the United States, in 1980. Quiroga had fled torture in Chile. His cofounder, psychologist Ana Deutsch, had fled Argentina's Dirty War, during which her family had been tortured. Leaders like Quiroga and Deutsch taught clinicians about torture as a lived experience. Their passion, bravery, witness, and resilience showed that healing was possible and that leadership, even under arduous circumstances, was necessary.

In 1978 the International Rehabilitation Council for Torture Victims (IRCTV) was established in Denmark.[9] Today, it operates a treatment center, seeks international funding for the care of torture survivors, publishes research, does antitorture advocacy, assists with asylum petitions, and trains staff at 162 member centers around the world. In 1985 the Center for Victims of Torture (CVT) in Minneapolis started with a domestic rehabilitation program and now has developed broad domestic and international programming for advocacy and rehabilitation.[10]

In 1984 the UN's Convention against Torture and Other Cruel, Inhuman or Degrading Treatment or Punishment asserted the duty of each nation to compensate and rehabilitate torture survivors: "Each State Party shall ensure in its legal system that the victim of an act of torture obtains redress and has an enforceable right to fair and adequate compensation, including the means for as full a rehabilitation as possible. In the event of the death of the victim as a result of an act of torture, his dependents shall be entitled to compensation."[11] In 2013 the WMA belatedly endorsed the right of rehabilitation for torture survivors and the work of the treatment centers.[12] Although it is difficult to study the effect of rehabilitation owing to scant funding, cultural and personal diversity, small sample sizes, and the attendant inability to randomize or do multivariate analysis, treatment centers decrease psychological symptoms and enable survivors to become economically productive members of society.[13]

As the rehabilitation centers' clinicians treated survivors, they discovered evidence-based ways to detect, assess, and treat torture-related injuries.[14] They learned how to correlate survivors' accounts of abuse with their injuries. For example, CT scans found a unique crushing of the rim of neck vertebrae bones in some persons who said that an electric cattle prod had been forced into their mouth and discharged against the back of the throat. The cattle prod had caused neck muscle spasms that in turn caused vertebrae to curve and slam against each other.[15] Clinicians also found tiny calcifications under the skin where electrical torture had been delivered.[16] This science improved the ability to use observations from autopsies and exams to prove that a person had been tortured. The forensic examination of photographs of tortured Syrians is one innovative way to use this science for human rights investigations.[17] The use of scientific findings has greatly improved the outcome of hearings to obtain asylum.[18]

James Jaranson and Michael Popkin describe the evolving relationship between the rehabilitation centers and the effort to end impunity for torture.[19] Rehabilitation center staff assist human rights monitors from organizations like the United Nations, the Red Cross, and Human Rights Watch. Centers provide translators, survivors, and local experts to examine prisoners and perform autopsies. The staff document the history and examinations of released prisoners and decedents. They provide photographs and x-rays of injuries. The centers' staff take great personal risks. Governments regularly shut down centers, as happened in 2017 to the Nadeem Torture Rehabilitation Centre in Egypt.[20]

DNA analysis has proved to be a useful forensic tool. Human rights organizations have advocated for or compiled DNA databases of families looking for "disappeared" loved ones.[21] DNA matches have identified bodies in mass graves. Matchers have also identified children who were stolen at birth by torturers who then killed their mothers (pseudonyms are used throughout this story):

> On October 6, 1978, Argentine soldiers kidnapped Rosa's daughter and son-in-law, Patricia and Jose. Patricia was eight months pregnant. The two were taken to a torture prison where fellow prisoners reported that Patricia gave birth to a son whom she named Rodolfo. Patricia and Jose were both disappeared.

The junta fell in 1983. Rosa searched for her grandson, Rodolfo, for more than twenty years. She was in contact with the Mothers and Grandmothers of the Plaza de Mayo, a human rights group composed of the families of disappeared prisoners who sought to learn the fate of their loved ones. It is estimated that five hundred babies were stolen by guards who did not want to kill the babies but who did not want the children to return to leftist homes where they would grow up to become enemies of the state that had killed their mothers. A prison doctor falsified the birth certificate to claim that the guard's wife was the birth mother.

In 1999, after the fall of the Argentine military junta, the Grandmothers of the Plaza de Mayo learned that a twenty-one-year-old man, Guillermo, might have been one of the stolen babies. Guillermo agreed to submit a blood sample. Forensic pathologists compared his DNA to samples in a DNA bank of grandmothers whose pregnant daughters had been disappeared. Guillermo matched to his grandmother Rosa, proving that he was the son of Patricia [NB: paraphrased from original technical text].[22]

As a result of this application of genetic science, guards were imprisoned for kidnapping and doctors were imprisoned for falsifying birth certificates (see chapter 11). The children faced wrenching choices. They had never known their birth families. They had been raised, sometimes affectionately, in families that were responsible for murder and kidnapping. After learning of the circumstances of their birth, some children returned to their birth families; others remained with the families that had raised them.

PHR is another kind of medical human rights organization. In 1986 Dr. Jane Schaller, its first president, described its mission as documenting human rights violations, advocating on behalf of colleagues who were endangered, developing a human rights curriculum for clinicians, and denouncing health professionals who participated in abuses.[23] With a modest budget, PHR pursued an extraordinarily broad set of activities, including supporting Chilean and Turkish physicians in danger for seeking to punish colleagues who assisted torture; deploying medical experts to exhume mass graves in Europe, Asia, and Africa to obtain evidence for criminal proceedings; using DNA analysis to reunite families in cases where military officials had stolen newborns from their murdered mothers; publishing reports on torture in many countries; promoting standards for collecting evidence of torture from medical examinations and autopsies (see chapter 9); and developing education materials for clinicians.

Dr. Robert Kirschner worked with PHR for several years. A forensic pathologist, Kirschner teamed up with Clyde Snow, a renowned forensic anthropologist (an expert in analyzing badly decomposed skeletal remains). Snow and Kirschner had identified bodies from several airplane crashes and serial killer cases in the United States before PHR recruited them in 1985 to excavate mass graves in Argentina to prove that specific units of soldiers had committed the mass murders.[24] Later, they applied their forensic archaeology to a grave containing 130 children murdered by the El Salvadoran Army. The two pioneered how to use site excavations to gather evidence for war and torture trials.[25] Kirschner was a tireless correspondent and a profound teacher. He was droll and sardonic. When asked on *Nightline* about a prosecutor who had criticized him for not talking like a bland medical expert, he commented, "I guess they thought I wasn't objective enough when I talked about exhuming one hundred and fifty bodies of civilians with their hands tied behind their backs."[26] Kirschner died of natural causes at sixty-one; his forensic methods were still a work in progress. Clea Koff's memoir of forensic anthropology in Rwanda, Bosnia, Croatia, and Kosovo gives a good sense of what this work is like.[27]

## The Istanbul Protocol

On August 10, 1993, twenty-nine-year-old Baki Erdoğan was arrested in Aydin, a city of 200,000 in western Turkey. The police held him incommunicado as a dissident. A prisoner in his cellblock later told of covering her ears as thuds and screams came from the room where police were interrogating Erdoğan. Eleven days after his arrest, police brought the battered Erdoğan to a hospital, where he soon died. The police concealed the death for two days. They did not let Erdoğan's father attend the autopsy. A government coroner and autopsy asserted that Erdoğan had died of a ten-day hunger strike. He was one of fourteen people to die during imprisonment in Turkey in the first ten months in that year.[28]

Members of the Turkish Medical Association (TMA) were skeptical of the official autopsy report and death certificate. The TMA successfully pressured for an independent autopsy. The second autopsy found that Erdoğan had died of blunt force trauma. At that time PHR and the TMA were working together to protect antitorture physicians from government reprisals.[29] The Erdoğan case took PHR's work in Turkey in a new direction.

In 1996 the Society of Forensic Medicine Specialists in Turkey, the Human Rights Foundation of Turkey, PHR, and the Danish IRCTV convened a task force to create an autopsy protocol as a guideline for coroners on how to systematically record injuries suggestive of torture. As discussed previously, torture often creates unusual injuries. Many of these injuries occur outside the internal organs that are the usual focus of autopsies seeking to determine the cause of death from disease. For example, suspending a person by arms that are twisted backward can cause unusual rotational tears of shoulder ligaments, which a coroner can find only by looking at the shoulder joints.

The task force's experts began with an older document, the Minnesota Protocol. In 1982 the United Nations heard testimony that pursuing extrajudicial homicide (i.e., death squad murders) in El Salvador was difficult because there was no validated way to autopsy the bodies.[30] Death squad murders can differ from ordinary homicides and battlefield deaths in how the bodies are found, whether there are signs of torture or binding, or how the fatal wounds are inflicted. The Minnesota Lawyers International Human Rights Committee partnered with pathologists to create a protocol to guide the systematic inspection of crime scenes and bodies. The 1991 Minnesota Protocol compiled evidence to use in trials to show that government forces were responsible for extrajudicial murders.[31] The protocol was successfully used during the examination of bodies found in mass graves left by the regime of Guatemala's former dictator, Gen. Efraín Ríos Montt.[32] In 2013 Ríos Montt was convicted for genocide and crimes against humanity. The Erdoğan case, of course, differed from the cases covered in the Minnesota Protocol. The Minnesota Protocol focused on death squad murders; Baki Erdoğan died of prolonged torture.

The task force produced the *Manual on Effective Investigation and Documentation of Torture and Other Cruel, Inhuman or Degrading Treatment or Punishment*, more commonly known as the Istanbul Protocol, for the city where the task force first convened.[33] The new protocol needed prominent endorsements to promote its authoritative standing in legal proceedings. In 1999 the United Nations endorsed the protocol for presenting forensic evidence. The United Nations High Commissioner for Human Rights published the protocol.[34] The UN Special Rapporteur on Torture routinely assesses whether local coroners who see deceased prisoners are familiar with the use of the protocol. PHR and IRCTV have programs for teaching how to use the protocol.[35] The WMA commended the protocol in 2003.[36]

The Minnesota and Istanbul Protocols show how clinical observations from rehabilitation centers and attentive coroners can be synthesized with legal advice to create robust tools to promote the cause of holding torturers accountable. The Minnesota Protocol was a major advance for investigating death squad murders, but it was not optimal for assessing torture. Baki Erdoğan's corrupted autopsy would have enabled officials to go free. A proper autopsy changed history. In June 2000 four police, a deputy security director, and an antiterrorism departmental director were convicted of torturing Erdoğan to death.[37]

New protocols are emerging. For example, the International Forensic Group has published a draft of how to assess medical records for torture.[38] Refinements of the Istanbul Protocol are needed to detect injuries from tortures that do not scar, such as waterboarding. Forensic protocols are powerful but insufficient if the will to hold torture doctors accountable is lacking. Even aside from holding torture doctors accountable before criminal courts or licensing boards, there are other notable forms of medical resistance to torture.

Sometimes this resistance takes the form of refusing governments' requests to collaborate with torture. In 2012 the Lebanese Order of Physicians said that physicians should refuse police requests to perform rectal examinations to assess for homosexuality; the Justice Ministry soon followed suit.[39] Chapter 3 describes the Australian medical community's resistance to the government's policy regarding refugee detention centers. In 2012 a court in Pakistan overturned an order to transfer a brave physician who resisted police pressure to prepare a false autopsy report.[40] In 2016 Egypt's Doctors Syndicate Assembly partnered with thirteen human rights groups to resist soldiers who were trying to pressure doctors to falsify medical records.[41] In 2017 the Kenyan Medical Association condemned forced anal examination despite directives from law enforcement officials; the court supported them.[42] In Tunisia the government banned anal exams in 2017, after physicians, with support from human rights groups, refused to perform them.[43] The Indonesian Doctors Association instructed its members to refuse to chemically castrate prisoners.[44] Islamic medical associations and medical associations in predominantly Islamic countries have taken a strong stance against physician participation in penal amputations, as discussed in chapter 6. For many years some Israeli physicians have refused to collaborate with torture, as, for example, in this incident of refusing to force-feed a prisoner on a hunger strike.[45]

Some physicians and medical human rights groups bravely document torture. The extraordinarily brave Zimbabwe Association of Doctors for Human Rights documented and decried torture in that unfortunate country.[46] The Egyptian Medical Assembly and Amnesty International supported the Nadeem Torture Rehabilitation Centre as it identified trauma caused by torture.[47] In 2017 a Ugandan torture victim rehabilitation center confirmed torture trauma as a cause of death despite government denials.[48] Physicians in Bahrain and Cameroon work with human rights advocates to document torture.[49] In the face of deadly reprisals, the brave Sudan Doctors' Syndicate details torture by its government.[50] The Turkish government asked the Human Rights Foundation's Torture Treatment and Rehabilitation Center to identify its patients[51] and fined Dr. Tufan Kose, who refused to surrender his patients' medical records because he feared that the police would use the records to pursue them.[52] These acts of bravery show that medical organizations and physicians, even in autocratic countries, can resist medical complicity with torture. C. S. Lewis's aphorism "Courage is not simply one of the virtues but the form of every virtue at the testing point" offers a way to assess both the professionalism of these physicians and the muted protests of the medical communities of Germany, Portugal, Spain, the United Kingdom, and the United States with regard to torture in their own prisons and by their own colleagues.[53]

# 10

# ORGANIZED MEDICINE'S CONDEMN AND ABIDE

In the decades after World War II, medical associations endorsed many declarations condemning physician complicity with torture. These declarations differed from typical medical "consensus statements" in that they did not present and assess research about torture's short- and long-term injuries to victims, loved ones, torturers, or civil society. Nor did they undertake to empirically rebut misconceptions that might incline a physician to abet torture, for example, the common misbelief that torture improves interrogation.

This chapter focuses on WMA statements, declarations, and resolutions against physician complicity with torture. Three reasons justify this focus. First, the WMA, a congress of 114 national medical associations, is the largest, most diverse, and most prestigious international organization speaking for the medical community. Second, as chapter 5 showed, the WMA was founded to address the stain of Nazi physicians' war crimes.[1] Its mission statement still affirms this view:

> TORTURE PREVENTION. Physicians: Key Actors in the Fight Against Torture.
>
> The World Medical Association (WMA) has a long-standing commitment to act for the prevention of all forms of torture and ill treatment. The WMA unequivocally condemns any involvement of physicians in acts of torture, whether active or passive, as a severe infringement of the International Code of Ethics and human rights law.[2]

Finally, most of the antitorture codes endorsed by hundreds of national and medical specialty associations use the WMA documents as templates.[3] This chapter shows that the WMA's condemnations of physician complicity with torture avoid taking on the necessity of holding torture doctors accountable and are silent on providing policies and procedures on how to do so.

WMA declarations against physician complicity with torture emerged in three phases. From the Nuremberg trial of Nazi doctors in 1946 until 1974, they focused on the general duties of physicians to prisoners. From 1975 to 1990 they focused on physician complicity with torture. After 1990 the WMA passed statements addressing specialized topics in medicalized torture. In 2009 Dr. Alfred Freedman and I synthesized the provisions of various WMA declarations on torture as of that date.[4] This chapter mentions concurrent developments in international law and UN resolutions that add historical context for the statements emerging from international medical associations.

The period from 1946 to 1974, the deep freeze of Cold War, begins with the Nazi doctors' trial and runs through the eve of the WMA's Declaration of Tokyo. It includes the WMA's aborted promise that torture doctors should be held accountable and the UN's 1948 Universal Declaration of Human Rights, which asserted the human right to be free from torture (see chapters 5 and 8). In 1949 the WMA, which had already acquiesced to the German position on not holding Nazi doctors personally accountable for their complicity in torture, passed the International Code of Medical Ethics, which asserted it was "unethical [for a physician to offer any] act or advice which could weaken physical or mental resistance of a human being." The code did not argue for holding transgressors accountable.[5] In 1949 the Third Geneva Convention Relative to the Treatment of Prisoners of War banned torture, to include medical complicity with torture: "Article 13: . . . no prisoner of war may be subjected to physical mutilation or to medical or scientific experiments of any kind which are not justified by the medical, dental or hospital treatment of the prisoner concerned and carried out in his interest."[6]

The UN's 1955 Standard Minimum Rules for the Treatment of Prisoners specified "model" medical care for any prisoner. Rule 32 contains three foreboding provisions:

1. Punishment by close confinement or reduction of diet shall never be inflicted unless the medical officer has examined the prisoner and certified in writing that he is fit to sustain it.
2. The same shall apply to any other punishment that may be prejudicial to the physical or mental health of a prisoner. . . .
3. The medical officer shall visit daily prisoners undergoing such punishments and shall advise the director if he considers the termination or alteration of the punishment necessary on grounds of physical or mental health.[7]

Rule 32 accommodated, for example, the widely accepted practices of having physicians certify prisoners as fit to undergo flogging or being placed in isolation (i.e., "the hole") and of monitoring the prisoners during the punishment.

In 1956 the WMA produced its Regulations in Time of Armed Conflict. Although the regulations did not reject Rule 32, they advanced medical ethics in two respects. First, they stated that it is "unethical for physicians to: (a) Give advice or perform prophylactic, diagnostic or therapeutic procedures that are not justifiable in the patient's interest; (b) Weaken the physical or mental strength of a human being without therapeutic justification; (c) Employ scientific knowledge to imperil health or destroy life."[8] This regulation starts to raise a barrier between physicians and the decision to impose flogging without barring a physician from monitoring a sentence of flogging while it is under way. Second, the regulations contain the remarkable statement that "medical ethics in times of armed conflict is identical to medical ethics in times of peace." This means that physician-soldiers (unlike soldiers who are not physicians) are not exempt from the core professional principle of medical beneficence as they care for enemy combatants or POWs.

## General Statements on Medical Complicity with Torture

From 1975 to 2002 the international community endorsed four documents relevant to physician complicity with torture. In 1975 the WMA passed Guidelines for Physicians concerning Torture and Other Cruel, Inhuman or Degrading Treatment or Punishment in Relation to Detention and Imprisonment (usually called the Declaration of Tokyo). Chapter 7 described how the BMA consulted Amnesty International's 1973 Paris Conference in developing this declaration.[9] The Declaration of Tokyo was updated in 2005, 2006, and 2016 from text given in chapter 4. The 2016 text condemns direct and indirect physician assistance with torture:

1. The physician shall not countenance, condone or participate in the practice of torture or other forms of cruel, inhuman or degrading procedures, whatever the offense of which the victim of such procedures is suspected, accused or guilty, and whatever the victim's beliefs or motives, and in all situations, including armed conflict and civil strife.
2. The physician shall not provide any premises, instruments, substances or knowledge to facilitate the practice of torture or other forms of cruel, inhuman or degrading treatment or to diminish the ability of the victim to resist such treatment.
3. When providing medical assistance to detainees or prisoners who are, or who could later be, under interrogation, physicians should be particularly careful to ensure the confidentiality of all personal medical information. A breach of the Geneva Conventions shall in any case be reported by the physician to relevant authorities.
4. . . . physicians have the ethical obligation to report abuses, where possible with the subject's consent, but in certain circumstances where the victim is unable to express him/herself freely, without explicit consent.

5. The physician shall not use, nor allow to be used, as far as he or she can, medical knowledge or skills, or health information specific to individuals, to facilitate or otherwise aid any interrogation, legal or illegal, of those individuals.

6. The physician shall not be present during any procedure during which torture or any other forms of cruel, inhuman or degrading treatment is used or threatened.

7. A physician must have complete clinical independence in deciding upon the care of a person for whom he or she is medically responsible. The physician's fundamental role is to alleviate the distress of his or her fellow human beings, and no motive, whether personal, collective or political, shall prevail against this higher purpose.

8. Where a prisoner refuses nourishment and is considered by the physician as capable of forming an unimpaired and rational judgment concerning the consequences of such a voluntary refusal of nourishment, he or she shall not be fed artificially, as stated in WMA Declaration of Malta on Hunger Strikers. The decision as to the capacity of the prisoner to form such a judgment should be confirmed by at least one other independent physician. The consequences of the refusal of nourishment shall be explained by the physician to the prisoner.[10]

Unlike Amnesty's Paris Conference document, all four versions of the Declaration of Tokyo are silent on holding torture doctors accountable. Thus, they continue the WMA's postwar position: condemn physician collaboration with torture in principle and abide by the impunity of torture doctors in practice.

In 1982 the UN adopted Principles of Medical Ethics, echoing the Declaration of Tokyo.[11] In 1984 the UN adopted the Convention against Torture and Other Cruel, Inhuman or Degrading Treatment or Punishment as the bedrock of antitorture international law.[12] (Chapter 3 discussed its definition of *torture*.) In 1988 the UN's Body of Principles for the Protection of All Persons under Any Form of Detention or Imprisonment defined "cruel, inhuman or degrading treatment or punishment" (a term of art in the Declaration of Tokyo) as "extend[ing] the widest possible protection against abuses, whether physical or mental, including the holding of a detained or imprisoned person in conditions which deprive him, temporarily or permanently, of the use of any of his natural senses, such as sight or hearing, or of his awareness of place and the passing of time."[13] This phrase can be used to assess sensory deprivation or solitary confinement. Finally, in 2002 the Rome Statute of the International Criminal Court barred torture and "subjecting persons who are in the power of another party to the conflict to physical mutilation or to medical or scientific experiments of any kind which are neither justified by the medical, dental or hospital treatment of the person concerned nor carried out in his or her interest, and which cause death to or seriously endanger the health of such person or persons."[14] The US signed the Rome Statute and then withdrew its signature.[15] The legally dubious effect of that withdrawal is outside the scope of this work.[16]

## Statements on Specialized Aspects of Medical Complicity with Torture

WMA statements have most recently focused on specialized aspects of physician complicity with torture. Six issues stand out: (1) a physician's duty to not force-feed prisoners who undertake hunger strikes, (2) the duty of a country not to grant a medical license to any immigrant physician who is charged with torture or other crimes against humanity in foreign countries, (3) a physician's duty to document and report torture, (4) a physician's duty to not perform rectal exams on allegedly gay men at the order of police, (5) a physician's duty to not participate in coercive interrogations, and (6) the duties of doctors who see prisoners developing mental illness in solitary confinement.

Physicians have the duty to respect the decisions of prisoners who hunger strike, either individually or as a part of a collective action to protest unjust sentences and brutal prison conditions or to promote political causes. Prisoners' hunger strikes are forms of political speech by persons whose civil liberties are curtailed by their imprisonment. Since World War II prison hunger strikes have occurred in many places, including Cuba, Israel, Northern Ireland, Turkey, and Guantánamo Bay.[17] Prison officials, usually asserting a duty to "save lives," often elect to discipline and then force-feed striking prisoners. They use a forced tube feeding technique whereby a tube is inserted into the prisoner's nostril and pushed down to the stomach so that liquid food can be administered. The technique of tube feeding prisoners often differs from the standard medical treatment in several ways: (1) the prisoner's body, limbs, and head are forcibly restrained into a fixed position; (2) the equipment may not be sanitary; (3) the tube may be large (e.g., if a stomach suction tube rather than a gastric feeding tube is used); (4) lubricants to ease the passing of the tube may not be used; (5) medically risky lubricants, such a lung-damaging oil instead of aqueous lubricants, may be used; (6) procedures to ensure the end of the feeding tube is in the stomach, rather than the lung, may be lax; (7) painfully and irregularly large volumes of liquid food may be administered, causing vomiting and possibly pneumonia; (8) the tube may be repeatedly removed and reinserted several times per day without justification; and (9) the feeding solution may contain material, such as pork, to which the prisoner has a conscientious objection. All nine of these are bad medical practices and, when implemented intentionally, constitute "torture or cruel, inhuman, and degrading treatment or punishment."

The ICRC affirmed prisoners' right to hunger strikes during the conflict in Northern Ireland of 1981. The ICRC and the UN stated that force-feeding hunger strikers constitutes "cruel, inhuman, and degrading treatment or punishment" and thus violates international law.[18] The WMA's 1991 Declaration of Malta and its Declaration of Tokyo assert that prisoners on a hunger strike should not be force-fed if they are competent, understand the medical effects of fasting, and have not been coerced to hunger strike by other prisoners.[19] No physician has been punished for force-feeding a prisoner in any WMA member country, including Cuba, India, Turkey, and the United States.[20] To my knowledge, the WMA has not censured any member medical association that grants impunity to physicians who force-feed hunger-striking prisoners.

Physicians indicted for torture and other crimes against humanity should not be able to continue to practice medicine (and evade prosecution) if they immigrate to a new country. In the 1990s it was discovered that several physicians who had been indicted were licensed to practice in Europe. In 1997 the WMA passed the Statement on the Licensing of Physicians Fleeing Prosecution for Serious Criminal Offences, which stated, "A physician who perpetrates [torture, war crimes, or crimes against humanity] . . . is unfit to practice medicine." It urged national medical associations "to ensure that physicians against whom serious allegations of participation in torture, war crimes or crimes against humanity have been made are not able to obtain licenses to practice until they have satisfactorily answered these allegations." It urged medical associations to "inform the appropriate licensing authorities of information they receive regarding physicians against whom serious allegations of participation in torture, war crimes or crimes against humanity have been made and should encourage the licensing authorities to take appropriate actions to ensure that such physicians have satisfactorily answered these allegations before granting them licenses to practice." This is the first WMA appeal to delicense doctors for crimes against humanity since 1948, as discussed in chapter 5. France revoked the hospital privileges of Dr. Charles Twagira, who fled a life sentence for participating in the Rwandan genocide.[21] France also dismissed Dr. Eugene Rwamucyo, another participant in the Rwandan genocide, from his hospital post.[22] The United Kingdom, in contrast, did not act against its Rwandan physicians.[23] The United Kingdom suspended the medical license of Dr. Mohammed Al-Byati for one year for complicity with torture in Iraq (see chapter 12).

Physicians have the expertise and duty to keep accurate medical records and to report torture to authorities within or outside government who can act on such reports. During the war on terror, which began in 2001, US physicians failed to report the torture of prisoners in Iraq, Afghanistan, Guantánamo Bay, and various CIA black sites (see chapter 13), yet reporting these abuses to human rights groups would not have endangered these doctors. In 2003 the WMA's Resolution on the Responsibility of Physicians in the Documentation and Denunciation of Acts of Torture or Cruel or Inhuman or Degrading Treatment asserted that medical expertise makes physicians "privileged witnesses" to torture, that they should know how to recognize and document injuries caused by torture, and that they should report their findings to government officials when possible or to human rights groups when government authorities are unresponsive or dangerous. This resolution asserted that the failure to document and report might constitute collaboration with torture. Then the WMA, which writes medical codes of ethics, mysteriously retreated: "There is no consistent and explicit reference in the professional codes of medical ethics and legislative texts of the obligation upon physicians to document, report or denounce acts of torture or inhuman or degrading treatment."[24] Actually there is. The reference may be found in the WMA's Declaration of Tokyo: "A breach of the Geneva Conventions shall in any case be reported by the physician to relevant authorities."[25]

In many countries, police ask doctors to perform rectal or vaginal examinations on arrested persons purportedly to assess whether the detained person is homosexual or is an unmarried woman who has been sexually active (see chapter 6). In 2017 the WMA passed its Resolution on Prohibition of Forced Anal Examinations to Substantiate Same-Sex Sexual Activity, which states physicians should not perform anal examinations to assess homosexuality. This resolution is profoundly defective in that it inexplicably fails to address the practice of virginity examinations on imprisoned women.[26] Again, the WMA made no call for holding doctors accountable.

Physicians should not abuse psychiatric knowledge by assisting a government's effort to break prisoners down for interrogation or other purposes. The modern concern about misuse of psychiatry dates to unfounded fears of the efficacy of Communist brainwashing and the Soviets' abuse of psychiatry during the Cold War. In 1996 the World Psychiatric Association (WPA), a congress of national associations of psychiatrists, published the Madrid Declaration on Ethical Standards for Psychiatric Practice, which stated, "Psychiatrists shall not take part in any process of mental or physical torture, even when authorities attempt to force their involvement in such acts."[27] After the war on terror scandal in which psychiatrists and especially psychologists oversaw abusive interrogations (see chapter 13), the WPA issued the more detailed Declaration on Participation of Psychiatrists in Interrogation of Detainees.[28] This declaration does not address accountability.

Physicians must not monitor the deteriorating mental health of prisoners who are in solitary confinement without intervening to stop or report the abuse of a prisoner. Although the problem is global, the United States has a far larger number and percentage of prisoners in isolation than does Europe.[29] Determining when the prisoner's conditions of confinement are so brutalizing as to constitute torture requires complex analysis. The first issue is defining when solitary confinement is so severe that it becomes torture or cruel, inhuman, or degrading treatment or punishment. The second issue is defining when physician oversight of prisoners in solitary confinement becomes complicity with torture. Because this book focuses on torture doctors, I am not going to delve into the intricacies of the first issue, but I will comment on the second.

Sentencing a prisoner to solitary confinement can fill the criteria for torture. First, solitary confinement differs from the brief use of emergency isolation to address an imminent threat of harm to self or others. Solitary confinement is imposed by a government official, often at the discretion of wardens who are unconstrained by due process or appeal. Sentences to solitary confinement are often routinely renewed, sometimes for years or decades. Research finds that solitary confinement causes severe harm to mental health because people need human companionship to maintain a sense of self, space, and time and to avoid regression and descent into depression.[30] Solitary confinement can intensify the suffering imposed by imprisonment to a degree far exceeding an ordinary prison sentence. The UN Special Rapporteur on Torture has endorsed the Istanbul Statement on the Use and Effects of Solitary Confinement: "When isolation regimes are intentionally used to apply psychological pressure on prisoners, such practices become coercive and should be absolutely prohibited."[31] The rapporteur has reported the following conclusions about solitary confinement:

> i.e. physical isolation in a cell for 22 to 24 hours per day, . . . may amount to cruel, inhuman or degrading treatment or punishment and, in certain instances, may amount to torture. . . .
>
> The weight of accumulated evidence to date points to the serious and adverse health effects of the use of solitary confinement: from insomnia and confusion to hallucinations and mental illness. The key adverse factor of solitary confinement is that socially and psychologically meaningful contact is reduced to the absolute minimum, to a point that is insufficient for most detainees to remain mentally well functioning.[32]

Numerous human rights groups define and condemn prolonged solitary confinement as torture.[33]

In 2015 the United Nations updated its Standard Minimum Rules for the Treatment of Prisoners to create the Mandela Rules.[34] By changing the definition of "lawful sanctions" within the Standard Minimum Rules, the Mandela Rules effectively amended the UN's Principles of Medical Ethics, which excused physicians from responsibility for "pain or suffering arising only from, inherent in or incidental to, 'lawful sanctions' to the extent consistent with the Standard Minimum Rules for the Treatment of Prisoners."[35] These excerpts from the Mandela Rules define the problem for physicians who see prisoners in solitary confinement:

> Rule 45: (1.) Solitary confinement shall be used only in exceptional cases as a last resort, for as short a time as possible and subject to independent review, and only pursuant to the authorization by a competent authority. It shall not be imposed by virtue of a prisoner's sentence [NB: this bars the routine placement of death row prisoners in solitary confinement]. (2.) The imposition of solitary confinement should be prohibited in the case of prisoners with mental or physical disabilities when their conditions would be exacerbated by such measures. . . .
>
> Rule 46: (1.) Health-care personnel shall not have any role in the imposition of disciplinary sanctions or other restrictive measures. They shall, however, pay particular attention to the health of prisoners held under any form

of involuntary separation, including by visiting such prisoners on a daily basis and providing prompt medical assistance and treatment at the request of such prisoners or prison staff. (2.) Health-care personnel shall report to the director, without delay, any adverse effect of disciplinary sanctions or other restrictive measures on the physical or mental health of a prisoner subjected to such sanctions or measures and shall advise the director if they consider it necessary to terminate or alter them for physical or mental health reasons. (3.) Health-care personnel shall have the authority to review and recommend changes to the involuntary separation of a prisoner in order to ensure that such separation does not exacerbate the medical condition or mental or physical disability of the prisoner.

In 2014 the WMA endorsed the Statement on Solitary Confinement, which generally conformed to the Mandela Rules:

9. The physician's role is to protect, advocate for, and improve prisoners' physical and mental health, not to inflict punishment. Therefore, physicians should never participate in any part of the decision-making process resulting in solitary confinement.
10. Doctors have a duty to consider the conditions in solitary confinement and to protest to the authorities if they believe that they are unacceptable or might amount to inhumane or degrading treatment.[36]

The WMA's statement bars physicians from participating in decisions to impose solitary confinement but does not specify a duty to document or report declines in the mental health of patients in solitary confinement. It is silent on whether the physician should report violations—such as of the Mandela Rules requirement that solitary confinement should not last more than fifteen days— whether it is for death row prisoners, whether the prison should be staffed for medical visits every day of the week, or whether the sentence to solitary confinement should be subject to independent review. It is silent on holding physicians accountable for complicity with torture or cruel, inhuman, or degrading treatment or punishment as the prisoner's mental health disintegrates during medically monitored solitary confinement.

Many physicians caring for the more than eighty thousand prisoners in solitary confinement in the United States are not in compliance with the Mandela Rules (including those who see prisoners in supermax prisons).[37] Typical prison practice is for physicians to briefly note observations about mental health. There is no validated instrument to assess the deteriorating mental health of prisoners who are held in isolation. The physician-patient relationship of a person in solitary confinement resembles that of physicians who monitor flogging, i.e., the clinician signs off on the continued imposition of the punishment until and unless a catastrophic psychosis or suicide occurs.[38] This is now becoming an issue in the prison inspections carried out by the UN Council on the Prevention of Torture, as shown, for example, in its report on Croatia.[39]

From time to time the WMA expresses concerns about torture in specific nations, such as Iran or Uzbekistan.[40] It resolved that the Zimbabwe Medical Association should advocate more vigorously on behalf of human rights and "report its progress from time to time," and it reaffirmed that resolution a decade later.[41] And yet the WMA continues to hold such national medical associations as members in good standing even though human rights reports show that medically abetted torture is continuing. The WMA occasionally speaks out against singular events, such as when it condemned Saudi Arabia for sentencing a dissident to one thousand lashes under medical supervision.[42] It took a similar position on behalf of a physician prisoner of conscience in Egypt.[43] These case appeals are commendable; however, although it has issued a statement condemning physician participation in forensic anal exams of gay men, the WMA has not issued a general position on the widespread practices of medical complicity with flogging or punitive amputations. From time to time the WMA also expresses solidarity with doctors who refuse to collaborate with torture, per its Declaration of Tokyo and Declaration of Hamburg.[44]

As an international organization, the WMA is in a better position to advocate for holding torture doctors accountable than many of its individual member national medical associations, some of which are constrained by being located within autocratic nations. In 2009 and 2011 the WMA seemed to be inching toward supporting accountability for torture doctors. In 2009 it urged "national medical associations . . . to investigate any breach of these principles by association members of which they are aware."[45] In 2011 it encouraged its member national medical associations "to investigate accusations of physician involvement in torture that were reported to it from reputable sources" and said it would "encourage and support the National Medical Associations in their calls for investigations by the relevant special rapporteur (or other individual or organization) when the National Medical Association and their members raise valid concerns."[46] The WMA has not acted to tangibly advance these statements. It has not

1. acted on its 1948 position to "undertake to expel from our organization, those members who have been personally guilty of the crimes referred to above" and to endorse "judicial punishment of such crimes";
2. compiled, endorsed, and published procedural guidelines and case books to serve as a template for medical boards or national medical associations for hearing cases against doctors who are alleged to have tortured;
3. called on its member national medical associations to develop policies and procedures for encouraging medical licensing bodies to (a) investigate allegations of physician complicity in torture and cruel, inhuman, or degrading treatment or punishment; (b) determine

appropriate punishments; (c) and refer credible allegations of illegal acts to government agencies or human rights organizations (the WMA could further require its members to regularly submit their policies and procedures for confidential inspection by the UN Special Rapporteur on Torture and the ICRC);

4. established procedures to audit and assess the performance of its member national medical associations' compliance with number 3, noting that a national medical association that does not undertake this task may be censured as institutionally complicit with torture or cruel, inhumane, or degrading treatment or punishment;

5. established a secure web portal to solicit and enable persons to report allegations of physician complicity with torture to the UN Special Rapporteur on Torture or other human rights groups for investigation or established policies and procedures for receiving and processing complaints about torture;

6. established an indexed public archive of reports by the UN and prominent human rights groups describing doctors assisting torture; and

7. established a public archive of records of completed actions holding doctors accountable by medical associations or licensing boards in order to educate the global community that accountability is possible and to serve as a reference for organizations as urged by the BMA in 2001.[47]

The WMA's unwillingness to promote policies and procedures to actively promote holding torture doctors accountable is disappointing as measured both by its origin in reaction to the horror of Nazi medical crimes and by its international stature. It is fair to conclude that the WMA's passivity in this regard makes it part of the infrastructure of impunity for torture doctors.

# PART IV

## THE DAWN OF ACCOUNTABILITY

# 11

# INNOVATIONS

There have been sporadic attempts to hold torture doctors accountable even though medical licensing boards, professional associations, and governments leave the vast majority undisturbed. It is useful to think of the attempts to hold torture doctors accountable as arising from three transformative events: (1) the international campaign to pressure South Africa to hold physicians accountable for allowing torture victim Stephen Biko to die, (2) the protest of Western medical communities against the misuse of Soviet psychiatry, and (3) a cluster of cases in four South American emerging democracies. This chapter discusses these three events. Chapter 12 follows the ensuing spread of proceedings against torture doctors to additional cases and countries.

The 1975 court-martial of Greece's "orange juice" doctor, Dimitrios Kofas (chapter 8), could have marked the beginning of the effort to bring torture doctors to justice. However, human rights activists saw Kofas as simply one among many junta officials, and the records of that time do not highlight his medical position.[1] The medical community ignored the Kofas case altogether until a decade later, when it was commented on in the context of criticisms of the human rights abuses committed by Soviet psychiatry.[2]

## South Africa and the Murder of Stephen Biko

Shortly after Kofas was sent to prison, the 1977 torture murder of South Africa's antiapartheid activist Stephen Biko became an international cause célèbre. The shunned apartheid regime of South Africa was in the midst of a brutal endgame that continued for seventeen more years until it fell in 1994. During this time hundreds of doctors monitored floggings, oversaw torture, falsified medical records and death certificates, and labored to create biological and chemical weapons.[3]

Stephen Biko, an antiapartheid activist and former medical student, was arrested on August 18, 1977. The police brutally tortured him for three weeks. On September 7 he suffered three massive blows to his head and became delirious.

93

Dr. Ivor Lang, a police surgeon, briefly examined him and falsely noted that nothing was wrong. The next day Lang and Dr. Benjamin Tucker decided to send the shackled prisoner to a local hospital, where a spinal tap found that blood was oozing from his brain. The clearly abnormal test result was recorded as "normal" in the medical record. Tucker saw the semicomatose Biko three days later, on September 11. Lang and Tucker loaded the naked man into the back of a Land Rover and sent him 750 miles to a hospital without medical records or the abnormal spinal tap results. Biko died shortly after he arrived at the hospital.[4] Asked how he felt about the death, the minister of police brutally replied, "[It] leaves me cold."[5]

Human rights groups from inside and outside South Africa demanded justice for the murder. The WMA refused three times to accept a complaint against the doctors who neglected Biko.[6] The politics were complex.[7] The Medical Association of South Africa (MASA), which was dominated by the pro-apartheid South African medical profession, had withdrawn from the WMA in 1976 because it had felt political harassment for its physicians' role in torture and for the health disparities caused by apartheid. The WMA and AMA engineered a campaign to reinstate South Africa into the WMA. The campaign succeeded because the AMA pressured the WMA to allocate voting shares in rough proportion to members' financial support of that organization. The AMA, mumbling support for its South African colleagues, cast its bloc of thirty-six votes to reinstate South Africa over the outraged objections of many African members.[8] In 1982 the racially integrated National Medical and Dental Association (NAMDA) formed in protest of the segregated MASA.[9] In 1984, in an effort to rehabilitate its damaged reputation, MASA invited the WMA to hold its annual meeting in Cape Town, and the WMA accepted. NAMDA, in collaboration with many international human rights organizations, subsequently put enough pressure on the WMA that it had to move its meeting to Brussels, a humiliation that increased pressure on South Africa to address the complaint against the Biko physicians.[10] South Africa's courts and its licensing board continued to stonewall. South African human rights advocates, including some doctors, sued to force the South African Medical and Dental Council, the licensing board, to address the Biko doctors' negligence.

In 1985, eight years after Biko's murder, a South African court ordered the South African Medical and Dental Council to hold a hearing on the Biko doctors. The council eventually reprimanded Lang. By that time Tucker was within a year of retirement. The council suspended his license for three months, a penalty that was not to begin for two years—after his planned retirement.[11] The government compensated Biko's family.[12] The principal soldier who tortured Biko and lied to the Truth and Reconciliation Commission died of lung cancer, a broken man with PTSD.[13] After apartheid fell, the South African medical community apologized for the profession's general role in apartheid-era torture but rejected a proposal to convene a medical truth commission to look at the role of doctors in neglecting and overseeing torture.[14] NAMDA and MASA merged in 1998, after apartheid had ended.[15]

The Biko affair put a human face on a modern victim of torture doctors. It showed how a powerful configuration of medical, governmental, and cultural forces worked to protect torture doctors from accountability. The WMA's post-Nuremberg promise that torture doctors would be held accountable was dead and gone. The AMA, which had ardently proclaimed that physicians must not torture, actively worked against stigmatizing MASA or South Africa for failing to hold the Biko doctors accountable. The Biko affair seemed to show that accountability for torture doctors would be advanced by human rights activists rather than by medical organizations or the criminal justice system.

## Soviet Psychiatry

Valeriy Tarsis's 1965 autobiographical novel *Ward 7* awakened the West and its psychiatric community to the role of Soviet psychiatrists in suppressing dissidents (see chapter 6).[16] Tarsis's novel spurred human rights activists to interview dissidents who had been abused by psychiatric maltreatment. Those interviews revealed Soviet physicians as state agents who diagnosed dissidents with a nonexistent disease—sluggish schizophrenia—and then committed them to hospitals where the captive dissidents were abused with drugs that injured brains and caused disorientation, muscle spasms, coma from hypoglycemia, and even death. Beginning in 1971 the World Psychiatric Association (WPA) faced many calls to censure, suspend, or expel the Soviet Union's All-Union Society of Neuropathologists and Psychiatrists, to the enormous displeasure of the Soviet government.[17]

Western medical associations mobilized on behalf of Dr. Anatoly Koryagin, a Soviet psychiatrist whose paper describing Soviet psychiatric torture was published in the prestigious British medical journal *The Lancet* in 1981.[18] As Koryagin put it, "I can't be silent when people are kept in psychiatric hospitals for their political beliefs."[19] In 1981 the Soviet Union sentenced Koryagin to twelve years in prison, where he was tortured with psychotropic drugs and force-fed. Medical associations in Europe and North America made high-profile appeals on his behalf. That advocacy protected Koryagin and eventually secured his release from prison and deportation to the West. In 1983 the Soviet All-Union Society of Neuropathologists and Psychiatrists resigned from the WPA in an attempt to preempt WPA sanctions.[20]

The Soviet scandal showed that censure by global colleagues can make a medical society in a nation with torture doctors defensive. I cannot comment on whether this censure had the effect of decreasing mistreatment or medicalized abuse of dissidents. It did, however, show that concerted advocacy by international medical societies could protect an endangered physician of conscience. Yet the pressure on Soviet psychiatry never aimed to hold any individual Soviet torture doctors accountable. Unlike in the Biko case, the pressure in the Soviet case focused on Soviet leadership and psychiatric institutions.

## South America

The most extraordinary innovation in holding physicians accountable for torture was continental in scale. Beginning in 1980 Uruguay, Brazil, Chile, and Argentina collectively held approximately sixty doctors accountable for complicity with torture. One can surmise why these four countries undertook the unprecedented and roughly simultaneous process of pursuing their torture doctors. First, they emerged from vicious military juntas at approximately the same time. Argentina's Dirty War regime ended in 1983. Brazil's junta ended in 1985, the same year that Uruguay's junta lost power. In Chile, Gen. Augusto Pinochet's regime ceded power over the years 1988 to 1990.[21] Second, the four countries shared a continent and the largely mutually intelligible Iberian languages of Spanish and Portuguese. Third, they had similar Western European, Christian, and Latin American cultures with similar concepts of social justice. Even so, other South American nations that emerged from fascism did not imitate these four in the pursuit of torturers. Even within Brazil the effort to punish torture doctors seems to have been confined to two provinces. I am not aware of any collective work of history of these four countries in relation to torture doctors. Most academic articles focus on a single nation or briefly note anecdotes from several nations. Scholarship on the cross-border personal and institutional relationships that made these four countries leaders in prosecuting torture doctors would be fascinating.

Uruguay's military rule was brutal. Its Doctrine of National Security led to preventive repression against alleged atheists and Communists. There was wholesale imprisonment; a tenth of the population emigrated. As civil society became possible, the Uruguayan Medical Association took the leadership role in holding torture doctors accountable. The association affirmed the United Nations' 1955 Standard Minimum Rules for the Treatment of Prisoners and the WMA's Declaration of Tokyo, barring physician complicity with torture (see chapter 10). It convened a medical ethics court. The powerful Defense Ministry barred its physicians from testifying at civilian medical hearings and blocked the association's access to medical records from prison medical facilities.[22] Leaders of the Uruguayan Medical Association received death threats during the hearing of Dr. Eduardo Saiz Pedrini in 1984. The association had expelled Pedrini for falsely certifying that an imprisoned physician had not died of torture.[23] The junta allowed Pedrini to continue to practice as a military physician until it lost power in 1985. After 1989, when it became possible for the association to function openly, it received complaints against nearly eighty physicians, and it expelled thirteen for neglecting prisoners injured by torture or for creating medical records and death certificates to conceal torture: Hugo Díaz Agrelo (expelled in 1989), Vladimir Bracco (1989), José Pereyra Garay (1989), José Mautone (1989), Mario Sarusua (1989), Nelson Fornos Vera (1989), Elías Nassiffe (1989), Nelson Marabotto (2000), Salomon Cizín (1999), Juan Antonio Riva Buglio (2000), Arturo Dini Olivera (2000), and Marsicano Rosa (2000).[24] The association found neglect and falsifying records to be impeachable breaches of medical ethics, not law. The expulsions revoked the physicians' licenses to practice in a civilian capacity, but the government found ways to allow many of them to continue to practice.[25]

The Federative Republic of Brazil is fifty times larger and sixty times as populous as Uruguay. Because it is so much larger, after the junta had fallen in 1985, Brazil could not emulate Uruguay's centralized model for addressing the problem of torture doctors through one national medical association. Furthermore, it took decades for Brazil's government to confront the junta's bloody history. Brazil did not even charter its National Truth Commission to compile evidence of torture and disappearances under the junta until 2011. The commission did not report until 2014.[26] Thus, it is not surprising that the Federal Council of Medicine left the issue of torture doctors to state councils. In 1985 the twenty-six states ranged in size from São Paulo, with 35 million people, to Roraima, with 300,000. The Medical Councils of São Paulo and Rio de Janeiro received complaints alleging that at least 110 physicians had collaborated with torture; the two councils opened hearings against forty physicians.[27] The state councils' work was enormously advanced by their receptivity to meticulous documentation collected by human rights groups, especially Nunca Máis (Never Again) and the Catholic Archdiocese of São Paulo.[28] The São Paulo Medical Council forthrightly rejected pleas to let history lie, stating, "Amnesty is only legitimate for benefiting the victims of torture. It may not be used to protect torturers."[29]

The state medical councils' hearings were obstructed and complicated by amnesties, overturned convictions, and the natural deaths of some defendants during the prolonged process.[30] Bureaucratic appeals set aside sanctions that had been properly imposed. To protect the former junta's torture doctors, the government enacted a law stating that military physicians were accountable to health departments within the armed forces rather than to the state councils. This did not halt the councils' proceedings but did prevent them from revoking the licenses of physicians who worked for the former junta. The councils' potential sanctions ranged from confidential censure to public censure to temporary suspension or revocation of a license. Most of the accused and, of course, all of those who were never accused escaped punishment.

The effort to end medical impunity for torture in Brazil was inconsistent. Councils abandoned some cases because of the high cost of pursuing them. Death threats silenced some complainants. Records of hearings for dozens of cases simply end without any note on the disposition of the case. Brazil's second-most populous state, Minas Gerais, with about 15 million people in 1985, is more populous than the state of Rio de Janeiro. It is inconceivable that Minas Gerais was unstained by torture and torture doctors, but I cannot find that its council attempted to hold its torture doctors accountable. Neither did the other states as far as I am aware.

In 1980 Harry Shibata, a coroner, became the second physician after Nuremberg (Kofas from Greece being the first) to be punished for abetting torture. As director of the São Paulo State Forensic Medical Institute during the dictatorship, he had signed death certificates attributing deaths to "natural causes" without recording signs of torture and sometimes without even looking at the bodies.[31] As he described his work,

> Our function was purely technical. First thing in the morning we received bodies . . . and we performed autopsies to establish the cause of death. . . . Our task was only to establish the medical cause of death and not the judicial cause of death. . . . [It] is purely descriptive . . . all that is on the body is observed and recorded. Now, the interpretation of these lesions is something we cannot give. A hematoma [a pocket of blood under the skin] could be a spontaneous hematoma or it could be a traumatic hematoma. But we just describe the hematoma.[32]

Shibata's description of the work of a forensic pathologist is entirely alien to the purpose of an autopsy, which is to opine on the cause of traumatic injuries and to classify death as due to homicide, suicide, accident, natural causes, or, rarely (and usually with long-dead decedents), undetermined. Dr. Graccho Guimaraes Silveira brusquely offered this excuse for his false death certificates to the National Truth Commission, "We had forty to forty-five corpses for a shift, we had to do it in a hurry."[33] I cannot find any record of punishment for Silveira or Dr. Roberto Bianco, another coroner who appeared at the same National Truth Commission hearing.

Counting Shibata, I am aware of eighteen Brazilian physicians who were penalized from 1980 to 2002 for collaborating with torture.[34] Thirteen of the eighteen were coroners punished for falsifying death certificates: Frederico Ildelfonso Marri Amaral (censured, 1999),[35] Renato Sergio Lima Cappellano (license revoked, 2003), Pérsio José Ribeiro Carneiro (license revoked, 1996), João Guilherme Figueiredo (license suspended, 2002), Rubens Pedro Macuco Janini (license revoked, 2002), Irany Novah Moraes (license revoked 2000), Cypriano Oswaldo Mônaco (license revoked, 2000), José Manella Netto (lost license 1999), Abeylard de Queiróz Orsini (license revoked, 2002), and Antônio Valentini (license revoked, 2002). Walter Sayeg's license was revoked in 2002 for observing torture and further for falsifying death certificates. A council revoked Dr. José Antonio de Mello's license in 2002, and later a court revoked his pension and ordered him to pay damages to a victim's family for writing a false death certificate.[36] The reason for the large number of coroners was that these specialists damned themselves by signing the false death certificates.

Other torture doctors were not coroners. Ernesto La Porta had his license revoked in 1992 for abetting torture. In 1999 José Coutinho Neto France lost his license for overseeing the torture of eleven prisoners.[37] Ricardo Agnese Fayad had his license revoked in 1994 for complicity with torture but continued to work in military medical facilities.[38] A celebrated case involved two prominent psychiatrists.[39] Dr. Leão Cabernite's license was suspended and then revoked in 1992 for abetting torture. Cabernite was a psychoanalyst; his analysand at the time, Dr. Amílcar Lobo Moreira da Silva, was a sadistic torturer whose license was revoked in 1988 (see chapter 2). Although Brazil has taken steps to address medical complicity with torture during the junta, medical complicity with torture remains a deeply embedded practice.[40]

Torture was common during General Pinochet's iron rule in Chile from 1973 to 1990.[41] Physicians who were suspected of being against the regime were tortured. In the waning years of the junta's power, as in Uruguay and Brazil, the Medical College of Chile opened dialogues with international human rights groups.[42] The purpose of these relationships was to prepare to respond to torture survivors' needs for rehabilitation and to hold torture doctors accountable. Chilean physicians were acutely aware that some of their colleagues had died of torture. Early on the college received reports of about a dozen physicians who allegedly abetted torture, although human rights groups have since documented the roles of thirty to almost forty.[43] But I am able to trace the outcome in only nine cases.

Before and during Pinochet's rule, expulsion from the Medical College of Chile had the effect of revoking the medical license because college membership was a prerequisite for having a license. The government countered the college's expulsions of torture doctors by removing the requirement for college membership as a condition for having a medical license. This reduced the effect of college expulsion to moral censure. In this situation human rights groups, such as the Ethics Commission against Torture, organized public campaigns to denounce torture doctors, as is discussed later in this chapter.

The Medical College of Chile punished at least seven physicians.[44] Dr. Carlos Hernan Perez Castro oversaw the horrifying torture of a woman for which, in 1982, his license was suspended for a year.[45] Perez Castro was murdered shortly after he was expelled from the medical association; it is not known if this was in reprisal for torture. In 1986 Dr. Manfred Jurgensen Caesar and Dr. Luis Losada Fuenzalida were expelled for falsifying records and participation in torture.[46] In 1986 Dr. Camilo Azar Saba was suspended for six months for his involvement in the torture of a prisoner.[47] Dr. Victor Carcuro Correa was expelled from the college in 1987 for participating in torture.[48] The college also expelled Dr. Guido Felix Diaz Mario Paci in 1987 for participating in and attempting to cover up torture.[49] Vittorio Orvieto Teplitzky was expelled from the college in 2005 and then sentenced to prison for six years in 2008.[50]

In addition to the seven physicians punished by the college, at least two physicians (aside from Teplitzky) were criminally prosecuted. In 2001 Dr. Osvaldo "Tormento" Pinchetti, a doctor who oversaw torture, was sentenced to fifteen years in prison and freed on bond.[51] In 2010 José Maria Fuentealba Suazo was sentenced to seven years in prison for abetting the disappearance of a prisoner.[52]

Argentina took a different path from Chile, Uruguay, and Brazil. After the junta fell, the Argentine government promptly created a national commission to investigate the torture and disappearances carried out during the Dirty War of 1976 to 1983.[53] The Argentine Medical Association and the National Academy of Medicine of Buenos Aires remained silent.[54] Four years after the junta fell, it appeared that the medical community might rise to the task. In 1987 the medical faculty of Buenos Aires University held a public convocation on physician complicity with torture that was attended by more than two thousand people.[55] That convocation censured three doctors (Jorge Hector Vidal, Julio Ricardo Estévez, and Jorge Antonio Bergés) for violating the Hippocratic oath, the National Code of Ethics, and international ethics standards. The three physicians censured by the university assembly were eventually tried by criminal courts. In 1986, soon after democracy had been established, Bergés was sentenced to six years in prison, but he was released by a 1987 law that excused officials who claimed to have been acting under orders. He returned to medical practice.[56] In 1996, on the twentieth anniversary of the coup that ushered in the junta, two gunmen ambushed and critically wounded Bergés, who protected himself by using his wife as a shield. Two hospitals refused him admission before he was admitted and saved by Evita Hospital, ironically named for the former wife of Juan Perón, whom the junta that employed Bergés had overthrown.[57] In 2005, after the amnesty law had been revoked, Vidal was convicted for participating in numerous lethal tortures and sentenced to prison; his sentence was commuted to home imprisonment because of his poor health.[58] Estévez was indicted for commandeering a civilian hospital to use as a torture center, but he died before trial. Since then Dr. Carlos Ferreyra of Médicos con Memoria (Doctors with Memories) and Dr. Luis Justo have tried to spur the Argentine medical community to hold torture doctors to account.[59] In 2012 members of the National Commission of Bioethics resigned as a former justice minister who was accused of but avoided arrest for crimes against humanity was appointed to that body.[60]

Clinical facilities have occasionally acted where the Argentine Medical Association would not. In 1994 a torture survivor sought care for her child at a hospital and was shocked to recognize one of her former torturers, Dr. Néstor Ángel Siri. She reported him to a human rights group. The Buenos Aires minister of health dismissed him from his departmental directorship at the hospital but lacked the authority to revoke his license.[61] The Children's Hospital Association declared him a persona non grata because of his work in a torture prison and his noncooperation in clarifying the parentage of children born to disappeared women. He apparently continues to work as a clinician. As detailed in the introduction, Dr. Faustino Blanco Cabrera was sent to prison in 2006. He was released soon thereafter and returned to practice. In 2013 his background in torture was rediscovered. The hospital where he was working revoked his privileges. The province declared him a persona non grata, and a second trial sent him to prison for seven years.

After the junta the government granted amnesty to many torturers whom I have not tabulated because they were not convicted. Dr. Agatino Di Benedetto received amnesty but later faced an international indictment for genocide and terrorism. Eventually he was put on trial in Argentina, where the court found him to be insane.[62] The repeal of the amnesty law in 2005, two decades after the junta fell, cleared the path for criminal trials of torture doctors. Courts prosecuted some torture doctors. Obstetrician Dr. Jorge Magnacco falsified birth certificates and directly tortured. He had been identified and denounced by human rights groups. A demonstration at his home prompted his neighbors to ask him to move. He was arrested in 2001 and became the first physician to go on trial after amnesty had been revoked. In 2005 he was sentenced to ten years in prison and had two more trials and convictions. His sentences were combined into one fifteen-year sentence.[63]

In some prisons, guards called themselves doctors; the following cases involve bona fide physicians.[64] In 2010 Omar Ramon Capecce, Jorge Habib Haddad, and Raúl Eugenio Martin were imprisoned.[65] Alberto Arias Duval was indicted for about a hundred kidnappings (i.e., falsifying birth certificates to steal babies from persons who were murdered in prison as described later) and died during his trial in 2012.[66] In 2014 four physicians and a midwife were sentenced. Hilarión de la Pas Sosa was sentenced to twenty-five years in prison for torture.[67] Dr. Norberto Atilio Bianco and his midwife Luisa Arroche were sentenced to prison for involvement in kidnapping.[68] Omar Caram was fined and imprisoned for complicity with torture.[69] Carlos Octavio Capdevila was sentenced to prison for involvement in kidnapping, supervising torture, and murdering a prisoner with an injection.[70] In 2015 Dr. Vincente Ernesto Moreno Recale was sentenced to ten years in prison for directly supervising torture.[71] That same year Andres Leonardo Garcia Calderone received three years.[72]

A special aspect of medicalized torture in Argentina related to women who were pregnant at the time of their arrests.[73] The women were kept alive until close to term, and then delivery was either induced prematurely or carried out by C-section. The woman was then murdered, and her corpse was either dumped into the ocean or mass graves. Doctors (and occasionally, midwives) created false birth certificates saying that an official's spouse or relative was the baby's biological mother. Prison doctor Ricardo Lederer wrote a false birth certificate assigning parentage to his nephew and wife of a two-month-old infant who soldiers took when they arrested his mother. Thirty-two years later Lederer committed suicide when a DNA match between the grown child and a biological grandparent revealed the falsification. The nephew was sentenced to eight years in prison for kidnapping; his wife was sentenced to six years.[74] Dr. Julio César Caserotto was indicted on similar charges and died before a verdict was reached.[75]

In 2018, thirty-five years after the fall of the junta, the Argentine Catholic Church belatedly released more than a hundred baptismal certificates from the main prison where babies were taken from women who were then put to death.[76] During the junta the families of the disappeared pregnant women did not know what happened to the women or their unborn children. The kidnapped babies grew to middle age. It is fair to say that the church was part of the cloak of impunity for the doctors who assisted in the kidnappings and murders.

At least thirteen Argentine doctors have been convicted for criminal acts. Civil society censured or revoked medical privileges and rank as well. Others died before long-delayed indictments could result in verdicts. At least five died before a trial was convened. At least two were too ill to stand trial. At least one is in exile in a country that will not extradite him to stand trial. I will not name physicians who were acquitted as I cannot judge if those acquittals were just. The Fahrenheit Group maintains a dated list of about forty alleged torture doctors; a third of the forty are listed as escaping trial either by amnesty for persons working under military command or by a statute of limitations.[77] I have not been able to track all of those cases, but each of the cases that I have found confirm that report. I also identified cases that the Fahrenheit Group did not list. Medical torture continues in Argentina. In 2016 Dr. Fernando Nolberto Zaghis was given a suspended sentence for issuing a clean bill of health to a tortured prisoner whom he had not examined.[78]

In the previously discussed countries, a human rights tactic called "denounce," whereby groups accuse officials of human rights violations, often supplied the energy that led to formal accountability. In Argentina, Chile, and Uruguay, there are groups with names that capture their methods, such as Si No Hay Justicia, Hay Escrache! (If There Is No Justice, Denounce!).[79] Denounce groups compile dossiers on officials, including physicians, that include biographies and photographs of torturers and victims. These files summarize military careers as well as the histories of persons who were arrested and disappeared. When possible, other prisoners' accounts of what happened to the disappeared person in prison are included. The dossiers are often posted on websites that also display the officials' home and work addresses and telephone numbers. Denounces targeting physicians often cite "do no harm." The groups organize demonstrations that go to the alleged torture doctors' homes and offices and paste pictures of victims and painted condemnations on walls and streets. Denounce groups also seek policy reforms, such as repealing amnesties, statutes of limitations, and other laws that create impunity for torturers. Given that civil society (e.g., journalists, clergy, student leaders, intellectuals, and opposition political leaders) is the target of torture, torture is committed by governments, and that inaction by governments and medical bodies creates an infrastructure of impunity, it should come as no surprise that the denounce tactic is how civil society fights back.

At their most basic level, denounces express grief and anger at government torture officials who seem to be escaping accountability. Denounces are also an organizing tactic that seeks to spur courts and medical boards to impose formal accountability. This tactic works, as when South Africa was pressured to convene hearings against the physicians who were complicit in the murder of Stephen Biko. Finally, denounces are themselves forms of accountability that cause patients to leave torture doctors, hospitals to revoke privileges (as in the cases of Bergés and Siri), and neighbors to ask torturers to move out of neighborhoods or even into exile (see chapters 2 and 13). The Nazi torture doctor Hans Joachim Sewering was forced to withdraw from consideration for WMA president (chapter 6). The chasm between the humanity of medicine and the inhumanity of torture can engender violent reprisals. Dr. Carlos Hernan Perez Castro of Chile was murdered shortly after he had been expelled from the medical association, possibly in reprisal for torture. The Argentine physician Jorge Antonio Bergés was nearly assassinated for his complicity with torture.

The innovations discussed in this chapter opened the door to confronting torture doctors' impunity. Nevertheless, this chapter shows the tenuous nature of accountability. In most cases the medical community, either through national (Uruguay, Chile) or regional (Brazil) medical associations or a university-based medical school (Argentina), acted before courts. In Greece there was one court-martial. In South Africa, human rights advocates pressured a court to order the licensing board to act. Often governments move in to curtail the threat that its torture doctors might be held accountable, as we saw in Uruguay, Chile, and Brazil.

Licensing sanctions are, with few exceptions, the end of attempts to hold torture doctors accountable. Even where torture per se is not a crime, the elements of torture, such as assault, battery, rape, or homicide, are crimes. Falsifying a death certificate to conceal a homicide is being an accessory after the fact to a homicide. Argentina's imprisonment of doctors who had falsified birth certificates for being accessories to kidnapping illustrates this point. Confining the torture doctors' accountability to the level of professional misconduct, rather than criminal behavior, excludes the possibility of more severe sanctions imposed by courts, such as imprisonment, substantial fines, or restitution, or of the civil consequences of having a criminal record.

This chapter shows that only a small fraction of alleged torture doctors was held accountable in Chile, Uruguay, Brazil, and Argentina. In South Africa the trivial reprimands of the two doctors who were complicit in the torture murder of Stephen Biko are the numerator over a denominator of hundreds of physicians who abetted torture, including medically monitoring flogging (see chapter 6). It is hard to believe that Kofas was the only physician working in the Greek junta's torture prisons, although he is the only one named. The next chapter examines how accountability migrated to a global stage.

# 12

# GLOBALIZATION

This chapter tracks the few faint footprints of the quest to call torture doctors to account. The cases are difficult to find. The WMA does not ask its members to report cases of physicians who have been brought before licensing boards or courts for complicity with torture. Medical licensing board proceedings are often private. No national medical association that I am aware of issues annual reports on sanctions imposed on torture doctors. Trial court rulings are hard to find. Journalists treat hearings against torture doctors as important or unusual, but often they are censored or they do not follow cases that are quietly shelved. Even so, the newsworthiness of events to hold torture doctors accountable make them more discoverable than the torture doctoring itself, which has to be found during human rights advocates' visits (see chapters 4 and 6). I searched for references to reports of torture doctor trials and medical licensing board hearings in reliable news outlets, human rights organization websites, peer-reviewed articles, and United Nations reports from 1975 through March 2018.[1] Given a hint, I sought solid confirming reports.

The courts and medical boards of the present and former Communist bloc states (including the former Soviet Union and Warsaw Pact states, Czechoslovakia, Albania, Yugoslavia [and its successor nations], Cambodia, Laos, the People's Republic of China, Vietnam, and Cuba) have entirely failed to hold doctors accountable for torture. International human rights activists recently pressured Russia into prosecuting two doctors for abetting torture. In one case the government manipulated the statute of limitations and then delayed the proceedings to allow the potential for prosecution to expire.[2] The other defendant was acquitted after a short trial. This acquittal can be compared to Russia's usual prosecution success rate of greater than 99 percent.[3]

In Western Europe (i.e., Europe other than noted in the preceding paragraph), accountability is rare. Germany completely sheltered the Stasi torture doctors after reunification. I cannot find any sanctions relating to the not infrequent reports of abusive physicians in Portugal and Spain (see chapter 6). Italy punished several physicians for complicity with the 2001 police torture of protesters. Dr. Giacomo

Toccafondi was accused of beatings, insults, and violence and of cutting off the hair of women prisoners and keeping it as a trophy. He was sentenced to three years and six months in prison and fines, although all punishments were either suspended or reversed.[4] Drs. Aldo Amenta, Sonia Sciandra, Marilena Zaccardi, and Adriana Mazzoleni all received suspended sentences of two to three years for complicity with direct abuse and falsifying medical records.[5] Some civil cases against these physicians were mooted because of the statute of limitations. In 2013 Italy convicted five physicians and three nurses for the manslaughter of Stefano Cucchi, who died in 2009 of torture and neglect. A lengthy process of conviction, appeal with reversal, and appeal with conviction finally ended in an acquittal in 2016.[6] In view of the final verdict, I do not count the Cucchi case as a finding of accountability, although the process stigmatized all the defendants. I cannot find records of licensing actions in any of these cases.

Chapter 7 documents how a substantial, but uncounted, number of British physicians abetted torture during the colonial wars of independence and the Troubles in Northern Ireland and abetted flogging in the United Kingdom. About forty British physicians were allegedly complicit in abusing war on terror prisoners. Of all these cases, the United Kingdom has held torture doctors accountable in only the two cases cited in chapter 7. It revoked Derek Keilloh's license in 2012 for complicity with a torture murder, and in 2014 it suspended Mohammed Kassim Al-Byati for complicity with torture in Iraq before he immigrated.[7] The United Kingdom allows an indicted war criminal from Rwanda to practice. The numerator for accountability is trivial in relation to the denominator of impunity.

Torture is widely practiced by military and police forces throughout Asia (defined as including the Middle and Far East and Turkey but excluding previously identified Communist states). Chapter 6 notes one survey found that three-fourths of India's physicians had seen a tortured person and one-seventh had witnessed torture.[8] In 2006 the licenses of three Indian physicians were suspended for mutilating genitalia and breasts and for chopping off hands during autopsies, apparently to conceal the identity of the victim of torture, an act that constitutes complicity in attempting to cover up torture.[9] In 2007 the Sri Lanka Medical Council's Professional Conduct Committee suspended Dr. W. R. Piyasoma's license for three years for "infamous conduct in a professional respect" for a superficial and inattentive examination of a tortured patient who then died.[10] Another Sri Lankan doctor was suspended for two years in approximately 2011 for abetting torture.[11] In Pakistan a doctor was arraigned for abetting torture in 2008, but that case has become untraceable and is not counted.[12] In 2011 two military doctors in Syria were banned from a hospital operating room for three months for abusing patients.[13] This kind of administrative sanction is hard to detect. In 2015 the Turkish Medical Association censured and fined a Dr. A. K. about $300 for failing to note and report torture.[14] Given the prevalence of torture in Asia, the rare reports of physicians being held accountable for complicity with torture again suggest that impunity is the norm.

Torture is widely practiced in Africa. It is extraordinarily rare for any physicians there to be held accountable for assisting torture. In 1990 the Egyptian Medical Association established a system for receiving and processing complaints against physicians for complicity with torture.[15] In 2012 there was a widely protested acquittal of an Egyptian army doctor who conducted virginity tests on imprisoned Egyptian women.[16] An Egyptian medical human rights society advocated for criminal prosecution and a professional inquiry by the national dental association against Hazem Farouk, DDS, for collaborating with torture. In 2014 Farouk was sentenced to prison for fifteen years.[17] Three Rwandan doctors who were also senior officials, Drs. Gérard Ntakirutimana, Clément Kayishema, and Eliézer Niyitegeka, were punished for genocide, as discussed in chapter 2. The South African medical board issued two mild sanctions against the doctors in the Biko case, as discussed in chapter 11.

In the Western Hemisphere the brief suspension of Dr. Chand in Guyana in 2009 (see chapter 1) is the only case that I can find other than those discussed in chapter 11. US institutions afforded complete impunity to all their physicians and psychologists for torture during the war on terror, although a court ordered the government to compensate a couple of victims of torture, as discussed in chapter 13.

How many torture doctors have been held to account? Since my focus is on clinicians who participate in torture, I set aside the six Serbian and Rwandan doctors who were senior government officials overseeing large-scale human rights abuses (see chapter 2). I would also exclude Dr. Bashar al-Assad of Syria, should he ever be held accountable for war crimes. Also in this category is South Africa's Dr. Wouter Basson, who was censured by the medical board for designing, deploying, and distributing chemical weapons; he was not charged with oversight of torture. Second, I do not count doctors who died while a trial was under way, whose cases were mooted by amnesties before a verdict could be reached, or who were acquitted, although this group would perhaps increase the number of cases of clinician torturers by severalfold. I also exclude physicians who were censured by hospitals, cities, or human rights groups without ever being punished in a criminal trial or by a licensing board. Anecdotal reports of such censures in Syria and in Argentina are described. Finally, I count only the first trial or license punishment of any physician in order to avoid counting any one physician multiple times for the same or related offenses. For example, chapter 11 notes that the Medical College of Chile expelled Dr. Vittorio Orvieto Teplitzky and that a court later sentenced him to prison. By these means, I have pared my count down to the number of individual physicians held accountable by medical licensing boards or criminal courts.

Courts or medical boards have formally held about eighty physicians accountable for complicity with torture since the Nazi doctors' trial. The cases were in Argentina (fourteen criminal convictions for complicity during the Dirty War plus one 2016 license suspension), Brazil (eighteen license sanctions, one of which included a court-levied fine, plus one medical board censure), Chile (seven license suspensions, including one prison sentence, plus two criminal convictions), Egypt (one criminal conviction of a dentist), Greece (one court-martial with a prison sentence), Guyana (one license suspension), India (three license suspensions), Italy (five criminal convictions), South Africa (one license suspension, one licensing board censure), Sri Lanka (two license suspensions), Turkey (one medical association censure and fine), United Kingdom (one license revocation and one suspension), and Uruguay (fourteen license sanctions). It is notable that licensing sanctions are much more common than criminal convictions. It is also clear from these numbers and the context of physician complicity with torture described in this book that only a minuscule percentage of torture doctors is ever formally held to account.

Figure 12.1 shows a time line of the licensing and court rulings holding torture doctors accountable. Again, duplicates are omitted. Cases are given in five-year intervals starting with Greece's 1975 court-martial of Dimitrios Kofas. The medical licensing actions of the innovating nations of Uruguay, Chile, South Africa, and Brazil dominate the next thirty-five years. One optimistic note is that after 2007 new precedents arose in an increasing number of countries outside the innovating countries discussed in chapter 11. Note that the most recent period considered, January 1, 2015, to July 1, 2018, is only forty-two months, not the full sixty months covered in the earlier periods.

The tally and the graph underrepresent efforts to hold alleged torture doctors accountable. For every physician sanctioned by a licensing board or sentenced

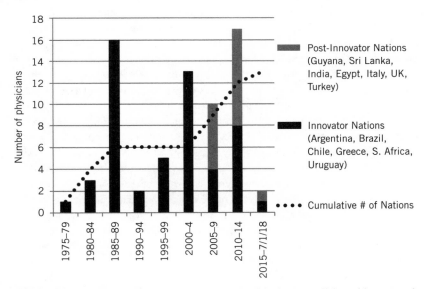

**FIGURE 12.1:** Number of physicians held accountable for complicity with torture by courts or medical boards, January 1975–July 2018

by a court, there were many more for whom the publicly announced start of a
proceeding was not followed by a final adverse ruling. Proceedings for many
denounced physicians were started but never finished. Absent final rulings, I did
not name them. I did, however, attempt to trace these starts. Some physicians
died, some were declared too ill to be tried, and some were granted amnesty after a
proceeding had been convened but before a verdict was reached. Some physicians
emigrated to escape a trial. Some proceedings simply faded into thin air.

## Reflecting on the Forms of Accountability

Criminal trials and medical licensing proceedings are very different forms of accountability. Because efforts to hold torture doctors accountable are in their infancy, an
enormous amount of scholarship is needed to understand how to most effectively
use these two types of accountability in various sociopolitical circumstances.

Courts punish crimes. In many countries torture, as defined in human rights
(i.e., the infliction of severe pain by an official), is not a statutory crime. However,
its component elements—threats, battery, rape, and murder—are crimes. Domestic courts prosecute those crimes rather than torture. For example, a doctor who
falsifies a death certificate to say that a person died of natural causes can be prosecuted for being an accessory to murder. Courts may sentence persons to prison
or house arrest. Prison sentences are usually a few years and are often suspended.
In some cases, such as the Cabrera case, there may be an irregular early parole
(see the introduction). Sentences are more severe in infamous cases that receive
public scrutiny, such as those of the Argentine doctors who falsified birth certificates for the babies of murdered women prisoners. Those doctors were charged
with abetting kidnapping because the birth certificates diverted children to other
families. I do not know of any domestic court that has imposed the death penalty on physicians who assisted torture. Governments shield physicians from the
collateral consequences of a trial. Legal costs seem to be paid in large part from
military budgets. Some government physicians continue to draw military stipends
or pensions after convictions. Governments often allow physicians whose licenses
have been revoked continue to practice, as we saw in Chile, Uruguay, and Turkey.

Courts in Argentina, Brazil, Guyana, Italy, South Africa, and the United
States have ordered compensation to be paid to victims or their families, as noted
throughout this book. Usually the government, rather than a torture doctor, pays.
Timor-Leste, Morocco, Sierra Leone, and Peru convened truth commissions that
memorialized abuses, set the stage for constitutional or legal reforms, and in some
instances, awarded reparations.[18] The United Kingdom recently paid reparations to the elderly survivors of torture by castration during the Kenyan fight for
independence.[19]

Medical boards have leverage over torture doctors because physicians are
licensed while they torture and they continue to work as licensed physicians when
they return to ordinary practice.[20] Nations have various structures for exercising

power over medical licensing. Some establish national or provincial boards, most with some degree of independence from the Ministry of Health. Some governments charter a medical association to grant and revoke a membership that is in turn a prerequisite for having a license. As we have seen, governments can change these charters to remove the association's power over licensing (see chapters 1, 11, and 14).

Medical licensing boards punish *unprofessional conduct* as defined by a medical practice law or regulation. Sometimes the standard of practice is specific, for example, the requirement to accurately complete death certificates. Other times the standard of professionalism can be an elastic concept. Aside from torture, licensing boards often hold doctors accountable for actions that are not against the law. For example, boards often punish physicians who have sex with patients because patients are seen as vulnerable in the asymmetrically powered intimacy of the medical relationship and sometimes because the sex is seen as a transaction by which the patient improperly obtains treatments or diagnoses. With regard to torture, licensing boards have punished unprofessional conduct that violates the Hippocratic precept "do no harm" or the WMA's Declaration of Tokyo, which bans physician complicity with torture. Board sanctions may be imposed irrespective of whether the licensee has been indicted, convicted, or acquitted for a crime. The Biko doctors, for example, were never brought before a court.

Medical boards have the power to revoke or suspend a license or to simply censure a physician. They may also require ethics training or restitution through public service, although I am not aware of such sanctions being imposed on a torture doctor. Revoking a medical license obviously has the potential of decreasing a physician's income, although some governments create ways for torture doctors to continue to practice even after a license has been revoked. As we have also seen, being identified as a torture doctor by a suspension or being denounced by human rights groups can become a professional stigma when a torture doctors returns to practice in civil society.

Dire physician shortages in torturing countries create dilemmas for licensing boards in their role as stewards of physician supply. There is not one ideal number of physicians per capita; globally, there is one physician for every 550 persons.[21] The Uruguayan Medical Association expelled torture physicians when it had one doctor for every 300 persons. The Chilean Medical Association expelled physicians when Chile had only one physician for every 1,700 persons, and the government changed the law so that expulsion from the association no longer cancelled a license. Egypt had one physician for 1,800 when it sent one dentist to prison for torture. Guyana had one for every 4,500 people when it briefly suspended Dr. Chand in 2009.[22] India, which held three physicians accountable for mutilating a torture victim's corpse, had one per 1,400. The scarcity dilemma becomes even more acute when the torture doctor has rare skills (e.g., surgery).[23] In addition, physicians may emigrate, decreasing the physician supply. Governments experience physician shortages as political pressure, and this might cause them to be reluctant to revoke torture doctors' licenses. There is a need to develop innovative forms of sanctions against torture doctors in countries with severe physician shortages.

The anecdotal nature of this data set does not permit conclusions as to what explains difference in how nations pursue torture doctors. Globally, impunity is by far the norm. Many factors seem to have some effect on pressuring for accountability. First, there must be human rights advocates seeking justice. These advocates may be domestic (e.g., Argentina's Mothers of the Plaza, who fought to hold those who disappeared their children accountable) or foreign (e.g., the campaign that pressured South Africa to hold Stephen Biko's doctors accountable). Second, it is helpful if the society allows domestic and international human rights advocates to collaborate. The Chilean Medical Association's relationship with Denmark's International Center for the Rehabilitation of Torture Victims mobilized specialized expertise. Third, given the difficulty and costs of investigations, it is helpful if domestic courts and medical associations find a way to accept evidence compiled by human rights groups. In the state of São Paulo, Brazil, the Medical Council accepted material from the archdiocese and Nunca Máis files in its proceedings against torture doctors. Argentina's medical association stayed far removed from a large human rights movement. Fourth, the government must allow licensing bodies to pursue torture doctors. In all but Argentina and Italy, licensing bodies seemed more able than courts to reach a finding against a torture doctor. Legal proceedings are slower than actions by active licensing bodies (perhaps because of their complexity, restrictive evidentiary standards, or capacity), and judicial systems seem quite reluctant to prosecute their own government's torturers.

The United States has every element favoring accountability. It has a vigorous human rights community that communicates with foreign colleagues, a free press, and the Freedom of Information Act for obtaining government files. It has a well-organized constellation of medical associations, licensing boards, and judicial bodies. It has an ample physician supply. And yet not one physician, pathologist, or psychologist who collaborated with torture was called to account for complicity with torture during the US war on terror. This record illustrates the final critical component needed to hold torture doctors accountable: the will to do so. The next chapter examines the US experience in more detail.

# 13

# IMPUNITY AND THE US WAR ON TERROR

On September 11, 2001, partisans of al-Qaeda attacked New York City and Washington, DC. As it justly retaliated, the Bush administration irrationally turned to interrogational torture, despite extensive research that had shown it to be worthless and counterproductive for obtaining intelligence (see chapter 3). This chapter focuses on how impunity was crafted for the various clinicians who abetted war on terror torture. It will only briefly note the large literature on the complicity of physicians and psychologists with war on terror torture.[1] The superstructure of impunity from federal prosecution or military courts-martial was created in three steps. First, President George W. Bush's CIA and Departments of Justice and Defense wrote many memorandums (often cutting and pasting from one to the next) that are commonly called the "Torture Memos."[2] These memos asserted that none of the countless domestic and international laws and treaties against torture, including the Convention Against Torture and the Eighth Amendment, which bars "cruel and unusual punishments," were applicable to judging US behavior. These memos laid the foundation for future defendants to claim that they acted in good faith. Building from the early memorandums, in 2007 President Bush signed an order with the Orwellian title "Humane Treatment of Al Qaeda and Taliban Detainees":

> None of the provisions of Geneva apply to our conflict with al Qaeda in Afghanistan or elsewhere through the world because, among other reasons, al Qaeda is not a High Contracting Party to Geneva. . . .
>
> I determine that the Taliban detainees are unlawful combatants and, therefore, do not qualify as prisoners of war under Article 4 of Geneva. I note that, because Geneva does not apply to our conflict with al Qaeda, al Qaeda detainees also do not qualify as prisoners of war. . . .

I hereby reaffirm the order . . . requiring that the detainees be treated
humanely and, to the extent appropriate and consistent with military necessity, in a manner consistent with the principles of Geneva.[3]

Second, the government tried to conceal the torture program by classifying documents and preventing prison inspections by the International Committee of the
Red Cross. And finally, when it became widely known that prisoners had been
tortured, President Barack Obama foreclosed the possibility of federal prosecution
or courts-martial as he declassified and released four more documents describing the torture program. He grounded the impunity of US torturers in the Bush
administration's torture papers:

> In releasing these memos, it is our intention to assure those who carried out
> their duties *relying in good faith upon legal advice from the Department of Jus-
> tice* that they will not be subject to prosecution. The men and women of our
> intelligence community serve courageously on the front lines of a dangerous
> world. Their accomplishments are unsung and their names unknown, but
> because of their sacrifices, every single American is safer. We must protect
> their identities as vigilantly as they protect our security, and we must provide
> them with the confidence that they can do their jobs. . . .
>
> This is a time for reflection, not retribution. I respect the strong views and
> emotions that these issues evoke. We have been through a dark and painful
> chapter in our history. But at a time of great challenges and disturbing dis-
> unity, nothing will be gained by spending our time and energy laying blame
> for the past.[4]

Obama's directive covered government disciplinary proceedings, courts-martial,
and federal prosecutions. To understand how government pathologists, clinical
physicians, and psychologists were protected from professional accountability, we
must look at how they were embedded in the interrogational torture program.

## Pathologists and Corrupted Death Certificates

The deaths of prisoners during war may result from torture, abuse, or neglect. To
promote monitoring of war prisons, Articles 120 and 121 of the Third Geneva
Convention Relative to the Treatment of Prisoners of War requires that prisoner
deaths be subject to medical inquiry and that death certificates be promptly sent to
an international organization, such as the ICRC.[5] These provisions aim to ensure
that deaths from neglect or torture become known promptly. The US government
and its pathologists systematically compromised reporting on deaths of prisoners.
For example, Gul Rahman was murdered at a CIA black site known as the Salt Pit
in Afghanistan in late 2002. His body was lost, and his death was concealed from
the public and his family for more than seven years.[6]

In the spring of 2003, photographs smuggled out of Abu Ghraib, a US interrogation center in Iraq, included one of smiling guards standing over a bruised body packed in ice in a body bag. That previously unreported death, of Mon Adel Al-Jamadi, led journalists to press the government about prisoners' deaths. The government released partial sets of death certificates that overrepresented natural deaths and concealed deaths by homicide and unsafe prison conditions. Al-Jamadi died during violent torture.

As human rights investigators obtained more documents, numerous anomalies were discovered. On March 30, 2007, Shibey Hamdan died after being shot at point-blank range with an assault rifle while he was in his locked cell; his cause of death was recorded as "indeterminate." Nagen Sadoon Hatab died as a soldier crushed his larynx by dragging him by his throat; the pathologist lost the specimen. Autopsies did not record fractures and bruises. Only brief notes refer to the deaths of an imprisoned child and a woman; there are no death certificates. In 2008 death reporting from prisons in Iraq and Afghanistan stopped altogether on the rationale that the prisons belonged to those nations even though US authorities decided when prisoners would be released.

In sum, US military pathologists falsified, misdated, or failed to file death certificates in a coordinated effort (judging from the synchronicity of false dating) to conceal prisoners' deaths.[7] The CIA's Office of Inspector General, the Armed Forces Institute of Pathology, and the individual pathologists failed to remedy the misreporting of death by torture. Obama's declaration of no "retribution" precluded disciplinary hearings, courts-martial, and federal criminal trials against them. American licensing boards, the American Academy of Forensic Sciences, and its *Journal of Forensic Science* all remained silent, even though the names of many physicians who signed corrupted death certificates are easily found.

## CIA Physicians, Waterboarding, and Rectal Feedings

As the torture program was being crafted in late 2002, Secretary of Defense Donald Rumsfeld appointed a working group to make recommendations on "enhanced interrogational techniques" (EITs). These counterresistance techniques were meant to coerce recalcitrant interrogatees. The working group reported "that the use of force was unnecessary to gain cooperation and was a poor interrogation technique given that its use produced unreliable information, damaged future interrogations and induced those being interrogated to offer [false] information viewed as expected in order to prevent the use of force." It cited many potential laws banning the techniques but deferred to the opinions in the Torture Memos. The working group further reported that the techniques departed from US doctrine and tradition, could be difficult to control, might undermine prosecutions, and might expose military personnel and contractors to prosecution. Rumsfeld ignored those cautions, authorized the EITs, and signed a provision stating that interrogators should ensure that "the detainee is medically . . . suitable (considering all the techniques to be used in combination)."[8] He authorized Defense Department personnel to use ineffective, traditionally illegal, and admittedly dangerous interrogations with physician monitoring. Physicians from the CIA's Office of Medical Services (OMS) were separately given the duty of monitoring that agency's use of EITs.[9] This section will discuss physician oversight of only two particularly cruel and dangerous techniques: rectal feeding and waterboarding.

CIA doctors oversaw "rectal feeding," a technique that causes interrogatees to suffer extreme pain.[10] The word *feeding* is preposterous in this context because neither the rectal nor colonic mucosa have any ability to absorb nutrients. Interrogators arbitrarily certified that the prisoner needed the "feeding." OMS physicians oversaw the insertion in a prisoner of a rectal tube customarily used in medical practice to decompress the colon or administer enemas. Pureed humus, nuts, or pasta was forced up the tube into the rectosigmoid colon, causing intensely painful distention. This procedure can cause rectal fissures that cause pain during bowel movements and take a long time to heal. Most of the time, rectal feeding, like waterboarding, scars the mind without leaving physical scars that forensic investigators can detect.

CIA physicians also oversaw the use of waterboarding interrogations. Waterboarding is a technique in which a prisoner is restrained on his back on a downward sloping board so that the head is lower than the feet. A cloth is placed over the nose and mouth to ensure that water cannot be blown off. Water is poured on the cloth and enters the nose to flood and block the upper throat, causing an intense feeling of being suffocated. A gasping prisoner inhales water into the lungs. CIA physicians recommended that waterboarding be done with medical saline instead of plain water to prevent inhaled water that was absorbed into the blood from diluting and dangerously lowering the blood sodium level (i.e., causing hyponatremia). No publicly published animal or human research supports the value of this improvisation. Physicians attended waterboarding sessions in case they were needed to perform emergency tracheostomies (i.e., cutting a hole into the windpipe) in the event a throat spasm blocked air from getting to the lungs.[11] It was recommended that waterboarding be applied no more than twice in one session, but soon the number rose to four applications per average session. Khalid Sheikh Mohammed was waterboarded eighty-one times in twenty-four hours; the medical officer was impressed by "how well KSM had withstood the experience."[12] The CIA chief of medical service's 2007 memo reflecting on coerced interrogations is a sad document. While complaining about the constraints of medical ethics and international law, he characterized the use of waterboarding as an "amateurish experiment" and went on to say there was "no reason at the outset to believe that it would be either safe or effective."[13] Yet in 1902 the United States had court-martialed Maj. Edwin Glenn for using the same "water cure" technique on prisoners in the Philippines.[14]

President Obama's declaration assured CIA physicians' impunity from government disciplinary actions and federal prosecution. In addition, unlike some of the pathologists who signed false death certificates, the names of the CIA physicians who oversaw waterboarding and rectal feeding are classified, putting them out of reach of medical licensing boards.

## Psychologists for War on Terror Interrogations

The embedding of psychologists in abusive Department of Defense war on terror interrogations started with memos between Guantánamo interrogators and the secretary of defense in 2002.[15] Gen. Geoffrey Miller at Guantánamo Bay created a committee of psychologists (and less commonly, psychiatrists) to oversee EITs. Behavioral science consultation teams at Guantánamo Bay and in Iraq reported to the intelligence system, meaning that the psychologists were not responsible for the prisoners' mental well-being. (Initially, the CIA's Office of Technical Services provided the psychologist oversight of CIA interrogations, but eventually it passed that role to OMS.[16]) BSCTs were operational by 2004.[17] BSCT members culled information from prisoners' medical records and from guards' observations to design a comprehensive set of biopsychosocial plans that aimed to break prisoners down to a hypothesized state of dependence (learned helplessness) in which the prisoner, contrary to fifty years of research, would surrender information.[18] Plans dictated the prisoners' experience during interrogation and in the cellblocks, including toilet privileges, sleep, meals, interactions with guards, and so on. BSCT personnel could direct that prescribed medical treatments be withheld to increase suffering or be used as incentives for cooperation. Not surprisingly, BSCT access to medical records and to medical manipulations caused prisoners to mistrust their health care providers to the further detriment of their well-being. BSCT plans were modified on the basis of interrogators' reports of a prisoner's response; modified approaches had names like "Fear up Harsh" or "Ego Down."

US military intelligence officials realized that they had to protect BSCT psychologists from being sanctioned for misconduct. In February 2005 military intelligence forged a covert collaboration with the American Psychological Association (APA) to create a cover for BSCT psychologists.[19] The APA created the Presidential Task Force on Psychological Ethics and National Security (PENS). Two-thirds of PENS members (as well as many additional observers during the meetings) were military intelligence personnel who had major roles supervising or conducting abusive interrogations. This stacked majority voted to bar members from taking notes and to keep the official minutes secret. PENS's mission was to protect BSCT psychologists from professional censure; the relevant science, ethics codes, or international laws were not allowed into the deliberations. The PENS report was tailored to accommodate the BSCT's policies and procedures. Intelligence personnel on the task force took the final draft of the report to senior Defense Department officials, who approved it. PENS then approved the report, and the Department of Defense appended it to BSCT policies.[20]

The PENS report said that psychologists (i.e., military intelligence psychologists) should not let multiple loyalties (such as a perceived professional responsibility to a prisoner's mental health) interfere with their primary duty to conduct the interrogation. Referencing PENS, the Department of Defense policy for psychologists stated,

> Psychologists and psychiatrists are not assigned to clinical practice functions but to provide consultative services to support . . . intelligence activities. . . . [The psychologist's job is] to provide psychological expertise to assess the individual detainee and his environment and provide recommendations to improve the effectiveness of intelligence interrogations. . . .
>
> The Ethics Code pertains only to a psychologist's activities that are part of their scientific, educational or professional roles: pertaining to the profession of psychology. The Code does not, therefore, have purview over the psychologist's role as a Soldier, civilian, or contract employee that is unrelated to the practice of psychology. For instance, the dictum for beneficence does not pertain to actions against the enemy in combat.[21]

The assertion that patient-serving ethics are suspended when a psychologist is working as an interrogational soldier was the green light for psychologists to work with abusive war on terror interrogations.[22] This assertion was also intended to offer a defense against future licensing actions for professional misconduct. That protection, as it happened, would not be needed.

The WMA's 1956 Regulations in Time of Armed Conflict (see chapter 10) states, "Medical ethics in times of armed conflict is identical to medical ethics in times of peace." This means that physician-soldiers, as distinct from soldiers who are not physicians, may not waive their duty of beneficence to enemies or enemy prisoners during war. With the PENS report, psychologists (who are admittedly not physicians) left medical ethics behind. Psychiatrists rejected the APA position. The president of the American Psychiatric Association succinctly stated, "Our position is very direct. . . . Psychiatrists should not participate on these BSCTs."[23] The Department of Defense stopped using psychiatrists and chose to work with psychologists instead. Neither the psychiatric association nor a licensing board ever took up the case of the psychiatrist who chaired the Abu Ghraib BSCT.

The most detailed description of what a BSCT did may be found in the log describing forty-nine days of the interrogational torture of Mohammed al-Qahtani at Guantánamo Bay in 2002.[24] Interrogators worked in shifts twenty hours a day. The BSCT suggested using a barking military dog, Zeus, to "exploit individual phobias"; using a swivel chair to prevent al-Qahtani from turning away from interrogators; and ignoring the prisoner's requests to go back to his cell between interrogations as his effort to gain control and sympathy. The BSCT oversaw the rotation of interrogation approaches with names like "Failure/Worthless," "al-Qaeda Falling Apart," "Pride Down," "Ego Down," "Futility," or "Guilt/Sin." Al-Qahtani was called "unclean" or "Mo" (for "Mohammed"), leashed, and made to "stay, come, and bark to raise his social status to that of a dog." He was made to growl at pictures of terrorists, forced to wear photographs of "sexy females," and ordered to study these photographs to identify whether various pictures of bikini-clad women were of the same or a different person. He was told that his mother and sister were whores. He was forced to wear a bra; a woman's thong was put on his head. He was told that he had homosexual tendencies and forced to dance with a male interrogator and stand naked in front of women soldiers. A female interrogator straddled him as he was held down on the floor, an approach called "Invasion of Personal Space" and "Futility." It was recorded that he became enraged when women soldiers instructed him on the Koran. He was not told, despite asking, when Ramadan was occurring. He was not allowed to pray in the manner of his faith. The interrogators kept the sleep-starved prisoner awake by playing loud music or white noise, yelling, or forcing him to stand, exercise, or dance. Interrogators performed an "exorcism" on the disoriented, sleep-deprived prisoner.

During a prolonged sleep deprivation, al-Qahtani was hospitalized for forty-two hours because his cell had been abusively cooled with an air conditioner (a technique called "Environmental Manipulation"). His body temperature fell to 95–97 degrees, causing his pulse to slow to a dangerous thirty-five beats per minute. Hospital doctors warmed him, corrected blood chemistries, and looked for a clot in a leg that was swollen because he had been kept strapped to a chair. Al-Qahtani was then hooded, shackled, put on a litter, and taken by ambulance back to the interrogation cell. Doctors and medics came to the interrogation room to monitor and approve the continuing abuse. On one occasion al-Qahtani was given "three and one-half bags of IV," which made him need to urinate. He was told to urinate in his pants, and he did so as he was tied down. Over two days in December, al-Qahtani gained eleven pounds after he had been given six bags of intravenous fluids of unspecified size. His pulse again slowed to forty-two beats per minute; an unnamed doctor consulted by phone said that "operations" could continue. There is no indication that the BSCT or medical personnel at the hospital protested or reported the abuse.

As word of PENS and interrogational torture leaked out, Psychologists for Social Responsibility (PsySR), Physicians for Human Rights, and other human rights advocates launched a vigorous denounce campaign against the APA's collaboration with military intelligence.[25] They researched declassified documents. They published letters and articles in professional journals and news media. "Withhold APA Dues" was a moderately successful program urging APA members to withhold dues until the organization retracted the PENs recommendations. PsySR members demonstrated and leafleted APA's national meetings and state chapters. It successfully lobbied psychology professional associations in Europe and North America to endorse ethics codes that rejected the APA's formulation of ethics. PsySR interrupted the APA's effort to obtain support for PENS from other professional groups, including torture survivor treatment centers. PsySR members ran for APA office. PsySR was able to get a resolution that would have asked psychologists to monitor the well-being and human rights of persons in military prisons before the membership for a vote. The Defense Department openly emerged to fight the resolution. In sum, PsySR prevented the APA from making the PENS debate disappear.

The APA finally commissioned an independent review of PENS, conducted by attorney David Hoffman. Jean Maria Arrigo, of the nonintelligence minority of PENS, had kept notes of and emails about the meetings. These notes and emails exposed the dominant role of military intelligence officials in drafting the PENS policy. In 2015 the extraordinary Hoffman report, based in part on Arrigo's contributions, detailed the collaboration between the APA and military intelligence and asserted that the APA's aim was to increase psychologists' opportunities in military and intelligence work.[26] Dr. Steven Behnke, the APA's ethics officer, was the public face selling the PENS report. During the drafting of the PENS report, he managed the APA's side of the collaboration with military intelligence. After the report had been released, he took a contracting job as a Defense Department intelligence contractor while he continued to serve as the APA's advocate. Hoffman discovered the conflict of interest, and shocked APA officials quickly fired Behnke. The APA apologized for the PENS debacle, rescinded the PENS report, and strengthened ambiguous policies. Senior and long-standing APA officers and board members resigned or retired. Jean Maria Arrigo was awarded the prestigious American Association for the Advancement of Science Scientific Freedom and Responsibility Award.[27] Some persons named by the Hoffman report are suing for defamation, among other things. So far a trial court and appeals court in Ohio have rejected the suit on jurisdictional grounds.[28] The denounce campaign against the APA focused on a professional society; it did not aim to hold individual psychologists accountable.

## Professional Accountability

In 2009 President Obama largely closed the possibility of federal or military prosecutions of or disciplinary actions against the architects or implementers of the war on terror torture program. Four options remained for holding the medical and psychological accomplices to abusive interrogations accountable: civil court suits, licensing board sanctions, and censure by professional societies or civil society.

After the names of two CIA psychologists who managed and oversaw interrogational torture had been inadvertently released when documents were declassified, civil suits were brought against them. The government tried but failed to prevent the public trial. The US settled the case and paid an undisclosed settlement to three torture victims just before testimony began.[29] The European Court of Human Rights held Poland, Lithuania, and Romania responsible for allowing the CIA to violate the European Union's prohibition of torture.[30] Each country paid about $100,000 to the two injured prisoners. Since the suits blamed the CIA rather than the psychologists overseeing the torture, the clinicians were, for our purposes, not held accountable for torture.

Licensing boards rejected complaints against three intelligence psychologists in Ohio, Texas, and New York.[31] In one example the APA and the State of New York found no cause for action against the psychologist who oversaw the al-Qahtani interrogation. In a curious coda the APA wrote to the Texas State Board of Psychologists saying that it would have expelled a psychologist who was the subject of a complaint if he had been an APA member.[32] However, the subject of another of those licensing board complaints was an APA member at the time of the abuse, and the APA elected to remain silent while the licensing board took no action. Identified physicians who managed force-feeding or a BSCT were not held accountable by licensing boards.

US medical associations sat on the sidelines as the scandal of medicalized torture unfolded. AMA journals, which are editorially independent from the AMA, did not join peers like the *Lancet, Surgery, Science, Medscape,* or the *New England Journal of Medicine* in publishing articles on US torture until the *Journal of the American Medical Association* ran an outside commentary in late 2005.[33] The BMA, the British Medical Foundation for the Care of Victims of Torture, and the American Medical Student Association called on the AMA to investigate and discipline physicians who had abetted the abuses.[34] The AMA simply asked the torturing Bush administration to investigate the claims itself.[35] The AMA and the American College of Physicians did not openly respond to UN and ICRC reports describing doctors' complicity with torture.[36] For example, they ignored this scathing indictment by the United Nations Commissioner on Human Rights:

> The Special Rapporteur has received reports, many confirmed by investigations of the United States military, that health professionals in Guantánamo Bay have systematically violated widely accepted ethical standards set out in the United Nations Principles of Medical Ethics and the Declaration of Tokyo, in addition to well-established rules on medical confidentiality. Alleged violations include: (a) breaching confidentiality by sharing medical records or otherwise disclosing health information for purposes of interrogation; (b) participating in, providing advice for or being present during interrogations; and (c) being present during or engaging in non-consensual treatment, including drugging and force-feeding.
>
> In sum, reports indicate that some health professionals have been complicit in abusive treatment of detainees detrimental to their health. Such unethical conduct violates the detainees' right to health, as well as the duties of health professionals arising from the right to health. The Government of the United States should revise the United States Department of Defense Medical Program Principles to be consistent with the United Nations Principles of Medical Ethics.[37]

American medical institutions were dead silent on holding the clinicians professionally accountable. The AMA's ethics officer said the AMA and national and international medical societies already had policies condemning torture and forbidding medical personnel from facilitating interrogation by withholding food or sleep deprivation: "That's not OK. We're not allowed to do that. . . . These policies need to be 'reiterated and disseminated.'"[38] In September 2004 the AMA and the WMA announced a course on the medical ethics of torture. The president-elect of the WMA (a former AMA president) demurely remarked that the timing of the new course "was not tied to reports coming out of Iraq or Afghanistan. . . . Because of things that are going on now, it's gotten more attention than it normally would have gotten."[39]

Even after the release of the shocking 2014 Senate report describing CIA doctors' roles in waterboarding and rectal feeding, the AMA remained aloof.[40] AMA president Robert Wah put it this way: "The AMA will continue to advocate that no doctor is asked to go against the ethics of the profession, to remind physicians of their ethical obligations, and to ensure that medical professionals are never involved in the abuse of detainees in U.S. custody."[41] In short, neither the AMA nor the WMA advocated holding US clinicians accountable for complicity with abusing prisoners, even though both institutions had once endorsed such a position in reference to the Nazi doctors.

By contrast the tiny medical human rights organization PHR promptly responded to the much-anticipated Senate report. It itemized the misconduct and called for accountability.[42] In response the *New York Times* editorialized,

> Health care professionals who engaged in or abetted torture should have their professional licenses revoked and, depending on the degree of culpability, be prosecuted criminally. . . .
>
> To ensure that result, Congress ought to enact legislation or the president ought to issue executive orders that explicitly prohibits all forms of torture and bars health professionals from direct involvement in interrogations. If Republicans feel the Senate report was biased, they should create a federal commission to investigate the role health professionals played in this barbaric undertaking.[43]

There were denounces against military and APA officials. Gerald Koocher, who became APA president in 2006, was a highly directive liaison to PENS. He abused dissenters on the task force and scorned human rights. In 2013 he became dean of the College of Science and Health at DePaul University. After the 2015 release of the Hoffman report, he survived a scathing public debate about his activities.[44] He left the editorship of *Ethics and Behavior*, a journal that he had founded. Russ Newman, a military intelligence psychologist who was instrumental in drafting the PENS report, resigned his position as provost and senior vice president for academic affairs at Alliant International University.[45] Bruce Jesson, a senior CIA interrogational psychologist, was forced to resign his position as a Mormon bishop.[46] Larry James was denied an interview for at least one academic job because of his role in the interrogations.[47] (James is quoted on human rights in chapter 2.) These kinds of censures are extremely poorly recorded.

The collaboration of US clinicians with torture became an international scandal. WMA members (i.e., national medical associations) knew that US clinicians had failed to report torture even though the Americans did not face risks remotely comparable to those faced by clinicians in other countries. As noted in chapter 10, the WMA passed a resolution declaring that doctors had a duty to document and report torture or cruel, inhuman, or degrading treatment to legal authorities and that the failure to do so might constitute complicity with torture.[48] The leadership of American medical associations and academies never demonstrated a degree of bravery even remotely approaching that shown by medical leaders of the Egyptian, Turkish, Sudanese, or other medical associations, as described in chapter 9 and elsewhere.

The US medical community lost a great deal by silently joining countries that confer impunity on torture doctors. It has forfeited its standing to speak with moral authority against medicalized torture in other nations. As Juan Méndez, the UN Special Rapporteur on Torture, put it,

> We had a sense of moral condemnation of torture that was truly universal. The nations that tortured denied that they did. . . . However, the example set by the United States on the use of torture has been a big drawback in the fight against such practice in many other countries throughout the world. I travel to parts of the world in my capacity of United Nations Special Rapporteur on torture and I can attest to the fact that many states either implicitly or explicitly tell you: "Why look at us? If the US tortures, why can't we do it?"[49]

# 14

# PROMOTING ACCOUNTABILITY

The news about torture is dismal and hopeful. Most nations torture.[1] Amnesty International found that half of the respondents from twenty-one countries fear being tortured if arrested.[2] A third of adults fleeing Somalia, Ethiopia, Eritrea, Senegal, Sierra Leone, Tibet, and Bhutan report having been tortured, although tortured persons are especially likely to flee.[3] Every nation has people, immigrants or native-born, who have suffered from torture. Although there is no global census of torture survivors, the number is surely many millions of men, women, and children. In 2000 the United States estimated that it is home to a half million torture survivors; other estimates are much higher.[4] On the hopeful side, torture appears to be declining. The Enlightenment and the abolition of slavery, peonage, and Christian ecclesiastical torture led to a significant reduction in torture in the eighteenth and nineteenth centuries.[5] Public spectacles of torture, such as whipping posts and breaking people on the wheel, are largely gone. Even over the last twenty years there seems to be a measurable decline in torture.[6] The debate about the prevalence of torture is somewhat independent of vigorous differences as to whether human rights institutions are ascendant or becoming obsolete.[7]

The suffering and disability caused by torture extend far beyond the immediate victims. Persons with post-torture physical disabilities and stress disorders are less likely to reach their full potential as successful parents, spouses, friends, workers, students, and participants in civil society despite some survivors' extraordinary openhearted resilience. Torture causes potential leaders of free societies, such as journalists, union leaders, and political leaders, to emigrate, depriving a country of their talents. If the disability, suffering, and death of torture were measured as they are for heart disease, torture would rank as one of the world's major public health crises. Even that measurement would overlook the adverse effects of torture on public health: for example, how torturing regimes suppress citizens from petitioning for drinkable water, safe industries, affordable housing, health care, and education.[8] Torture scarcely appears as a World Health Organization (WHO) priority. The WHO's Violence and Injury Prevention Program focuses on nongovernmental violence (e.g., automobile accidents or domestic violence), except for a small subsection on preventing violence against children that endorses preventing torture of women and girls (without mentioning boys or men).[9] The WHO's Mental Health Action Plan mentions that national health care systems should be accountable for addressing mental illnesses caused by torture.[10]

I must simply posit that holding torture doctors accountable is a worthy aspiration. It is unproven that the threat of accountability would decrease medical torture, induce physicians to report torture more regularly, or have any material effect in preventing regimes from recruiting the few doctors needed to abet or help conceal torture. Even so, there are five main reasons to hold torture doctors accountable. First, torture causes vast harms. Second, it is illegal under international law. Third, it is authoritatively and generally denounced as immoral. Fourth, the beast-healer contradiction of the torture doctor (see chapter 4) makes an effective meme for helping the public understand the evil of torture in the face of propaganda that presents torture as simply another tool of war. Fifth, doctors are "privileged witnesses" to torture in that their training and position puts them in a unique position to see and authoritatively assess and report torture.

The term *privileged witness* (like the word *sanction*) has several meanings, some of them opposites. As a privileged witness, a spouse may be ineligible to testify against his or her spouse in a court case. A privileged witness can also be a person with unusual expertise or proximity to an event such that their testimony is especially valuable. Physicians have, and can hone, the ability to identify, assess, and report on signs of torture. Chapter 9, "Healers for Human Rights," discussed how clinicians in centers for rehabilitating survivors of torture added to the forensic science of identifying injuries caused by torture. Although the Istanbul Protocol is a highly refined instrument for examining bodies, physicians with ordinary skill in the art of medicine know how to perform a history and examination to search for, assess, and record many torture-related injuries.

The issue comes to how the privileges of a physician will be applied to the problem of torture. In chapter 4, "What Is a Torture Doctor?" I defined a torture doctor as a licensed physician who applies knowledge and skills and his or her authorities to the service of performing or concealing torture. By contrast, therapeutic physicians use their knowledge, skills, and authorities to detect torture, heal the injuries, and expose the crime. These applications are in accord with the medical profession's duties of station and put the physician's knowledge, skills, and privileges on the side of health and human rights.

Chapters 7, 11, 12, and 13 review national experience in holding torture doctors accountable. They show that any given nation is at one of five stages according to how its courts or medical licensing boards hold physicians accountable for torture.

Stage I: Nations that entirely suppress discussion of holding physicians accountable for the abetting torture (e.g., North Korea, China, and many others).

Stage II: Nations that condemn physician complicity with torture in principle but do not punish doctors who do so (e.g., Israel, the Philippines, Portugal, the United States, and many others; NB: though not a nation, the WMA fits in this stage by neither holding its member associations accountable for tolerating torture nor promoting policies and procedures for its members to use in the service of ending impunity).

Stage III: Nations that have punished doctors for complicity with torture in symbolic cases (e.g., Egypt, Guyana, Great Britain, India, South Africa, Sri Lanka, and Turkey).

Stage IV: Nations or state provinces that have tried to systematically hold a set of torture doctors accountable (even though these efforts were vastly incomplete) in order to send a cultural message to their society (e.g., Argentina, Brazil, Chile, and Uruguay).

Stage V: Nations that systematically try to apply their justice systems to the task of holding torture doctors accountable (perhaps Italy).

The ability to rank these stages suggests that the agenda for human rights advocates, political systems, and medical associations should be to promote policies and procedures that lead nations to evolve toward Stage V. It also suggests a way to grade how well medical and legal communities are doing. The higher stages would disrupt the partnership between doctors and torturing regimes and hopefully foster a milieu in which physicians would be more likely to function as human rights monitors on behalf of prisoners at risk of torture and in furtherance of the public health benefits that accrue to societies without torture.

A government's torture doctors, the medical community, and civil society are in an unstable equilibrium. As we have seen, governments strive to provide torture doctors with impunity by excusing acts committed under orders or during national emergencies, requiring military screening of potential cases, and falsifying, classifying, or disappearing medical records. Some governments void the effect of sanctions levied by criminal courts or medical boards. Human rights advocates are threatened, sued for libeling officials or defaming the state, forced into exile, arrested, tortured, or killed.[11] The medical community has some power of licensing and has the ability to report honest assessments of injuries to domestic and international human rights advocates, who in turn can use their soft power to change government policies. International medical associations control where they hold conferences. The WMA, for example, moved a scheduled conference out of South Africa before the Biko doctors were held accountable. International medical associations can censure medical communities that are complicit with torture, as happened when Soviet psychiatry and US psychologists colluded with torture regimes.

Eleanor Roosevelt's "curious grapevine" of human rights activism arising from civil society has cracked through the hard pavement of impunity. David Forsythe describes how human rights are sometimes enacted as laws but how human rights can also be enforced as "soft law" by institutions of civil society.[12] Human rights organizations' denounces exemplify such "soft law" pressure. Oona Hathaway has shown that when civil society acts, it can push governments to reduce torture.[13] Transparency and accountability have reduced torture in the Republic of Georgia.[14] Although the medical community is often allied with the dominant political culture, civil society, in the struggle to assert betrayed human rights, often finds physicians' organizations more amenable to the pressure of "soft law," such as appeals to holding a doctor accountable for violating the ethic of "do no harm," than governments are responsive to attempts to get them to prosecute their own torturers. The medical community can be summoned with a "do no harm" ethic. Sometimes the medical community will respond with dissent, as described in chapter 9 and other parts of this book. Other times regional licensing boards, national medical associations, and hospitals will respond. In my view, medical associations' loosened ties from governments probably partly explain why their actions against torture doctors are more common than legal sanctions.

## An Infrastructure for Medical Accountability

In general, medical organizations are part of the societal infrastructure that is responsible for the impunity of torture doctors. Medical organizations have not set up policies and procedures to accept complaints. They routinely fail to process well-documented complaints, often relying on the disingenuous logic that the doctor has not been convicted by the torturing government. A complete lack of accountability is the norm; a symbolic response to celebrated cases is the fallback position. When medical organizations do punish physicians who have been complicit in abusing prisoners, they impose sanctions that are mild, brief, or suspended, and in any case these sanctions are far less severe than if a doctor had abused a person in his or her own basement. The profession's failure to hold torture doctors accountable is a structural failure to advance its core mission to promote clinical and public health.

It is possible to propose a medical infrastructure for holding torture doctors accountable. I shall only address the situation of medical licensing boards and associations.[15] I am not qualified to write on how to improve domestic courts' dismal record on prosecuting torturers. Any profession has four characteristic features: (1) educational institutions to convey specialized knowledge, (2) licensing that affirms qualifications and confers authority to do its work, (3) a code of ethics, and (4) self-policing institutions that uphold standards of competence and ethics.[16] I have not addressed the place of medical education in teaching how and why to detect and report torture. That small literature is easily found with academic literature search engines. Similarly, the small surveys of physician knowledge and attitudes toward torture are tangential to the focus of this book. I am not aware of evidence showing that education or sensitization of physicians will meaningfully constrict the supply of the few torture doctors who are needed to fill the desires of any regimes. There are ample numbers of antitorture declarations and ethics codes. So it is in self-policing where the medical profession is failing. Here are some thoughts on actions to be taken.

First, the WMA, national medical associations, and licensing boards must craft and endorse procedural guidelines to help medical licensing boards convene and conduct hearings. Lawyers, human rights groups, and medical leaders have the collective wisdom to write such material. A template has been published.[17] These guidelines might draw from medical licensing board case stories described in chapters 7, 11, and 12. The guidelines should

- discuss how licensing boards and associations might solicit, accept, screen, and investigate complaints;
- describe proper collaborations with reliable human rights organizations, including how to accept and verify information that they have compiled;
- define the complementary roles of courts and medical licensing boards in terms of usable evidence and burdens of proof; this definition should note that criminal convictions are not prerequisites for findings of unprofessional conduct (see chapters 11 and 12);
- note that a doctor's fear of being tortured as a justification for abetting torture is rarely justified (see chapter 2);
- discuss the possible sanctions that a board might impose (e.g., education, community service, censure, suspension of license, and revocation of the license);
- discuss possible appeals procedures; and
- provide a casebook describing typical kinds of misconduct and evidentiary problems and explaining how they were addressed, as well as identifying problems in setting sanctions.

However imperfect, the preceding material would be vastly better than the current void. It will be important that experiences in using these procedural guidelines be published and open for regular review so that the profession can improve them.

Second, the WMA should create and maintain a secure, encrypted web portal to enable human rights groups or national medical associations to report physician complicity with torture. The utility of such portals is well known to the human rights community.[18]

Third, the WMA should establish a public registry of cases that end in the application of criminal or board sanctions. This registry would serve as evidence of the WMA's national medical associations' efforts at ending the impunity of torture doctors. It would also demonstrate that accountability is possible and show how barriers can be overcome.

It will be impossible to craft a single punishment guideline for all medical licensing boards. Sanctions will vary according to the nature of the act, its celebrity, shortages of physicians, corruption, and many other circumstances. It may be possible to draft a range of sanctions and to list aggravating and extenuating circumstances that might justify a greater or lesser sanction.

It is conceded that few of a nation's torture doctors will be punished. Defendant physicians are selected for various reasons. Some, such as the doctors who oversaw the torture of antiapartheid leader Stephen Biko (chapter 11), are chosen because the incident causes intense public outrage. Others are selected because they are senior authorities. Some are selected because government actions (e.g., amnesties) have made only the pursuit of secondary defendants possible. Some are selected because of the atrocity of their work. The pursuit of accountability is inevitably an imperfect work of transitional and interstitial justice. Those imperfections do not excuse the norm of impunity.

The reason to pursue accountability for torture doctors is not simple vengeance. It is not about compensation, reparations, and rehabilitation for the victims, although these are worthy goals. Compensation or punishment cannot offset how deeply torture harms survivors, family members, the larger civil society, and the torturers themselves. To some degree, accountability is "restorative justice" as it burnishes medical communities that have been stained by complicity with torture. Ultimately, one may hope that the threat of holding torture doctors accountable may cause a few doctors to at least write their medical records and death certificates more honestly. Perhaps a few more might open quiet conversations with people in the human rights communities. Either step would let a bit more light into torture prisons. By such glimmers of truth, human rights advocates in civil society will more clearly see what needs to be done to prevent the gruesome work taking place in the gloom.

# APPENDIX

## Behavioral Examples of Torture Doctoring

A. Misuse of medical knowledge or skills
   1. The physician inflicts torture.
        A doctor directly tortures (Brazil,[1] Iraq[2]).
        A doctor beats a prisoner during a medical examination, etc. (Albania,[3] Syria,[4] Vietnam[5]).
        A doctor collaborates with the mutilation of prisoners (see chapter 6).
        A doctor designs programs to psychologically torture prisoners (see chapter 13).
        A doctor tries to obtain information from a prisoner under torture (Mauritania[6]).
        A doctor stocks rectal tubes knowing that they will be used to push semisolids into a large intestine to painfully distend the colon (United States[7]).
        A doctor tells guards that a prisoner requested medical care, and the guards beat the prisoner for that request (Mongolia[8]).
        A doctor selects, supplies, or suggests doses of drugs for intentionally and nontherapeutically causing coma or delirium and risking brain damage to a prisoner (Soviet Union in chapter 6; United States in chapter 13).
        A doctor administers drugs to a resisting person to facilitate interrogation (India[9]).
   2. The physician misuses medical knowledge or skills to abet torture by others.
        A doctor devises methods of torture that do not leave visible signs of torture (e.g., scars, healed fractures, torn ligaments, etc.) when the regime is susceptible to pressure from human rights advocates with forensic training.[10]
        A doctor proposes that interrogators use medical saline (instead of plain water) for a smothering torture (waterboarding) so that inhaled water does not dilute the salts in the prisoner's blood and cause cardiac arrest (United States[11]).
        A doctor trains guards to surgically cut off limbs (Sudan[12]) or blind prisoners (Iran[13]).

3. The physician misuses medical skills while providing treatment.

A doctor performs surgery on a wounded prisoner without pain medications to enable interrogation during surgery. Anesthesia is promised if the prisoner talks (Egypt,[14] United States[15]).

A doctor performs a hysterectomy on a person without telling her the purpose of the procedure and without obtaining consent (Uzbekistan[16]).

A doctor conducts virginity pelvic exams on naked women prisoners or rectal exams to assess for homosexuality in men as guards watch (see chapter 6).

A doctor devises and implements a protocol for nasogastric feeding by bolus that increases pain and that does not provide a standard of care to ensure that the feeding tube is in the stomach rather than the lung (United States[17]).

4. The physician misuses medical knowledge and skills to clear prisoners as fit for torture.

A doctor assesses and certifies a prisoner as medically fit for flogging (chapter 6), solitary confinement (chapter 10), or other forms of abuse or monitors and treats a prisoner so that the abuse may continue (Argentina,[18] Croatia,[19] Italy,[20] Jordan,[21] Kosovo,[22] Latvia,[23] Macedonia,[24] Myanmar,[25] Poland,[26] Portugal,[27] Qatar,[28] Spain,[29] Turkey[30]).

"Two other persons entered the room and introduced themselves as doctors. They examined me and checked me all over. One of them said to me that 'you must put up with it . . . there is nothing we can do' . . . [then electric shock torture]" (El Salvador[31]).

5. The physician misuses medical knowledge or skills to monitor prisoners being tortured so that the torture may proceed.

The doctor authorizes the continuation of torture (Argentina,[32] Soviet Union[33]).

During waterboarding, physicians and medics watch for signs of a potentially fatal throat spasm and are equipped to cut into the prisoner's throat to put an airway (a tracheostomy) in below the prisoner's closed larynx (United States[34]).

A tortured prisoner sees a doctor while guards are in the room. The physician says, "Did you get beaten up then, you crook?" Because he is still in the presence of his torturers, the prisoner states that he has not been beaten. The doctor allegedly replies, "Well go back and get your beating" (Brazil[35]).

A doctor resuscitates during torture to rouse prisoner for further abusive confinement (Mexico[36]).

6. Miscellaneous

A doctor mutilates bodies at "autopsy" to make the deceased less identifiable (India[37]) (NB: This is not torture because the victim is deceased, but it is complicity with torture and traumatizes the loved ones of the deceased prisoners).

B. The misuse of the authorities or duties conferred by a medical license.
  1. The physician misuses the authority to acquire and release medical materials for the purpose of torture.

Doctors allow a medical facility to be used for torture routinely (Albania,[38] Argentina,[39] East Germany,[40] Egypt,[41] Syria[42]).

A doctor manages and staffs a psychiatric hospital whose real purpose is the detention and medical abuse of political opponents (see discussion of former Communist countries in chapter 6; Georgia[43]).

A doctor stocks nasogastric tubes knowing that they are used to squirt acid into prisoners' stomachs (Soviet Union[44]) or to force-feed hunger strikers (Turkey[45]; see also United States in chapter 13).

A doctor allows interrogators to use a prisoner's personal medical records to design ways to abusively interrogate prisoners (see United States in chapter 13).

  2. The physician fails to create accurate medical records in order to abet torture.

A doctor at a psychiatric hospital gives dissidents false diagnoses of schizophrenia, signs papers to commit them, and writes orders to administer drugs that may cause severe short-term and permanent side effects (see former Communist countries in chapter 6).

A doctor falsifies the birth certificates of children born to murdered woman prisoners in order to assign the parentage to another military official and to remove the child from its biological family (see Argentina in chapter 11).

A doctor conducts a superficial examination and fills out a medical record that omits or minimizes injuries caused by torture or that falsely attributes injuries to a time when the person was not in custody (Bulgaria,[46] Iraq,[47] Israel,[48] Kyrgyzstan,[49] Macedonia,[50] Mexico,[51] Nepal,[52] Peru,[53] Romania,[54] Spain,[55] Sri Lanka,[56] Syria,[57] Tajikistan,[58] Thailand,[59] Turkey,[60] Ukraine,[61] Uzbekistan,[62] Venezuela[63]; see also Guyana in chapter 1). (NB: Sometimes this is done on official instruction or by official refusal to accept medical documentation of torture, in which case the issue becomes one of the duty to report torture [Mexico,[64] Morocco,[65] Togo[66]].)

A doctor falsifies death certificates to conceal or understate the severity of torture-related injuries or to delay the discovery of torture (Argentina,[67] Bahrain,[68] Burma,[69] Egypt,[70] India,[71] Iraq,[72] Malaysia,[73] Myanmar,[74] Peru,[75] Poland,[76] Romania,[77] Syria,[78] United States,[79] Uruguay[80]).

A doctor fails to complete a medical record at all (Algeria[81]; see also Guyana in chapter 1).

A doctor simply signs a medical record or death certificate for government use without seeing the prisoner at all (India[82]).

A doctor refuses to write a medical record for a tortured prisoner (Romania,[83] Tajikistan[84]).

3. The physician fails to undertake the treatment of a tortured person in a manner that abets the abuse.

> A doctor refuses to examine a tortured prisoner (Israel,[85] Kyrgyzstan,[86] Mauritania,[87] Mexico[88]).

> They took her to xx hospital, near yyy. . . . She told the doctor that she was raped (by officials). The doctor said, "That's not my job, I just check to see if you're sick" (Iraq[89]).

4. The physician fails to safeguard medical records for the tortured prisoners to use for their own interests.

> A doctor submits the medical record to the detaining authorities so that the prisoner and courts do not have access to its contents (Turkey[90]). A doctor loses or destroys medical records (Azerbaijan,[91] Bahrain,[92] Israel[93]).

5. The physician fails to report torture.

> The doctor fails to report treating a tortured prisoner up the chain of command or to human rights groups so that the interests of tortured persons can be protected. This includes situations where the doctor would be at no danger of reporting (Israel,[94] Jordan[95]) (NB: There are anecdotes of doctors not finding anyone willing to accept such a report).[96] There are also cases in which doctors are restricted from seeing prisoners because the doctors report injuries (Afghanistan,[97] Albania,[98] Cameroon,[99] Israel,[100] United States[101]).

6. The physician abets abusive research on prisoners that violates established research standards (United States[102]).

7. Miscellaneous

> The doctor knowingly or negligently promulgates nonscientific assertions about race, ethnicity, or the efficacy of torture that are used to support the use of torture (Germany[103]).

# NOTES

## Preface

1. Steven H. Miles, *Oath Betrayed: America's Torture Doctors*, 2nd ed. (Oakland: University of California Press, 2009); Steven H. Miles and Lisa Marks, eds., "United States Military Medicine in War on Terror Prisons," Human Rights Library, University of Minnesota, 2007, http://www1.umn.edu/humanrts/OathBetrayed/index.html.
2. Eric Stover and Elena O. Nightingale, eds., *The Breaking of Bodies and Minds: Torture, Psychiatric Abuse, and the Health Professions* (New York: W. H. Freeman, 1985).
3. British Medical Association (BMA), *Medicine Betrayed: The Participation of Doctors in Human Rights Abuses* (London: Zed Books, 1992).

## Introduction

1. "Faustino Blanco Cabrera, persona no grata" [Faustino Blanco Cabrera, persona non grata], InfoSur, August 22, 2013, http://infosur.info/faustino-blanco-cabrera-persona-no-grata/; "Condenan a médico de Cutral Co a 7 años de prisión" [Cutral Co doctor sentenced to 7 years in prison], Imneuquen.com, November 19, 2013, https://www.imneuquen.com/condenan-medico-cultral-co-7-anos-prision-n207067.
2. "Tenía una licencia, pero era juzgado por delitos de lesa humanidad" [He had a license, but was tried for crimes against humanity], *Rio Negro*, August 15, 2013, http://www.rionegro.com.ar/region/tenia-una-licencia-pero-era-juzgado-por-deli-LORN_1231582.
3. "Quieren declarer persona no grata medico Cutral Co" [They want to declare persona non grata doctor of Cutral Co], Lmneuquen.com, August 27, 2013, https://www.lmneuquen.com/quieren-declarar-persona-no-grata-medico-cutral-co-n198290.
4. Redacción Plan B, "Médico Torturador y Paciente Víctima se Encuentran en Consulta Psiquiátrica" [Torture physician and victim patient in psychiatric consultation], *Psiquiatrianet* (blog), November 5, 2013, http://psiquiatrianet.wordpress

.com/2013/11/05/medico-torturador-y-paciente-victima-se-encuentran-en
-consulta-psiquiatrica/.

## Chapter 1. Dr. Chand Sees a Burned Boy

1. Gaulbert Sutherland, "Several Cops Had Known of Teen's Torture Report," *Stabroek News*, December 9, 2009, http://www.stabroeknews.com/2009/archives/12/09/several-cops-had-known-of-teens-torture-report/.

2. Michael Jordan, "Medical Council Recommends That Doctor Be Suspended," *Kaieteur News*, December 13, 2009, http://www.kaieteurnewsonline.com/2009/12/13/medical-council-recommends-that-doctor-be-suspended/.

3. "Torture: Teen Experiencing Hell in Custody," *Kaieteur News*, October 31, 2009, http://www.kaieteurnewsonline.com/2009/10/31/torture-2/.

4. Michael Jordan, "Doctor Admits to Mistakes during Medical Council Meeting," *Kaieteur News*, February 1, 2010, http://www.kaieteurnewsonline.com/2010/02/01/doctor-admitted-to-mistakes-during-medical-council-meeting/.

5. "Medical Council Probing Police Surgeon's Treatment of Torture Victim," *Stabroek News*, November 17, 2009, http://www.stabroeknews.com/2009/archives/11/17/medical-council-probing-police-surgeon%E2%80%99s-treatment-of-torture-victim/.

6. Guyana Human Rights Association Executive Committee, "Minister of Health Makes a Mockery of Guyana Medical Council: GHRA," letter to the editor, *Catholic Standard*, April 30, 2010, 8, http://www.diocese.cc/upload/images/originals/30%20aprl%202010%20CSt.pdf.

7. Mahendra Chand, "Allegations about 'Callous Indifference' to Tortured Teen Completely Spurious," *Stabroek News*, November 14, 2009, http://www.stabroeknews.com/2009/opinion/letters/11/14/allegations-about-%E2%80%98callous-indifference%E2%80%99-to-tortured-teen-completely-spurious/.

8. Nirpati Persaud, "Dr. Mahendra Chand Has Been Very Kind to Us Shut-Ins," *Stabroek News*, March 17, 2010, http://www.stabroeknews.com/2010/opinion/letters/03/17/dr-mahendra-chand-has-been-very-kind-to-us-shut-ins/.

9. "Dr. Chand's Treatment of Torture Victim Leaves a Lot to Be Desired," *Stabroek News*, November 15, 2009, http://www.stabroeknews.com/2009/opinion/letters/11/15/dr-chand%E2%80%99s-treatment-of-torture-victim-leaves-a-lot-to-be-desired/.

10. "Medical Council Gives Doctor in Torture Teen Probe One Week to Respond to Findings," *Stabroek News*, December 8, 2009, http://www.stabroeknews.com/2009/archives/12/08/medical-council-gives-doctor-in-torture-teen-probe-one-week-to-respond-to-findings/.

11. Michael Jordan, "Doctor Fails to Respond to Medical Council," *Kaieteur News*, December 30, 2009, http://www.kaieteurnewsonline.com/2009/12/30/doctor-fails-to-respond-to-medical-council/; "Doctor Who Treated Tortured Teen Suspended for Two Months," *Stabroek News*, December 13, 2009, http://www.stabroeknews.com/2009/archives/12/13/doctor-who-treated-tortured-teen-suspended-for-two-months/; and Michael Jordan, "Medical Council Recommends That Doctor Be

Suspended," *Kaietur News*, December 13, 2009, http://www.kaieteurnewsonline
.com/2009/12/13/medical-council-recommends-that-doctor-be-suspended/.

12. "Teen's Torture . . . Ramsammy Awaits Revised Decision on Police Surgeon,"
*Stabroek News*, April 8, 2010, http://www.stabroeknews.com/2010/archives/04/08
/teen%E2%80%99s-torture-2/.

13. "Ramsammy Inaction over Sanction for Doctor in Torture Case a Travesty—
WPA," *Stabroek News*, February 7, 2010, http://www.stabroeknews.com/2010
/archives/02/07/ramsammy-inaction-over-sanction-for-doctor-in-torture-case-a
-travesty-%E2%80%93-wpa/.

14. "Torture of Teen: GPHC Awaits Word from Medical Council on Police Surgeon,"
*Stabroek News*, May 1, 2010, http://www.stabroeknews.com/2010/archives/05/01
/torture-of-teengphc-awaits-word-from-medical-council-on-police-surgeon/.

15. "Teen's Torture: Ramsammy Approves 'Censure' of Police Surgeon," *Stabroek
News*, April 28, 2010, http://www.stabroeknews.com/2010/archives/04/28/teen
%E2%80%99s-tortureramsammy-approves-%E2%80%98censure%E2%80%99
-of-police-surgeon/.

16. Leslie Ramsammy, Guyana Minister of Health, "Press Release—Dr. Mahendra Chand," news release, April 28, 2010, http://positiveguyana.wordpress.com
/2010/04/28/press-releases-press-release-dr-mahendra-chand/.

17. Twyon Thomas v. Attorney General (2011) 2010 No. 12-M, Demerara, High
Court of the Supreme Court of Judicature.

18. "Court Awards Tortured Teen $6.5M," *Kaieteur News*, June 18, 2011, http://
www.kaieteurnewsonline.com/2011/06/18/court-awards-tortured-teen-6–5m/;
and "$6.5 M Awarded to 14-Yr-Old Boy Brutally Tortured by Police," *Guyana
Chronicle*, June 18, 2011, http://guyanachronicle.com/65m-awarded-to-14-yr-old
-boy-brutally-tortured-by-police/.

19. "Gov't Clears Its Name in Promotion of 'Torture Cops,'" *iNews Guyana*,
January 29, 2015, http://www.inewsguyana.com/govt-clears-its-name-in
-promotion-of-torture-cops/; "Leonora 'Torture Cop' Kicked Out of Force,"
*Kaieteur News*, June 3, 2015, http://www.kaieteurnewsonline.com/2015/06/03
/leonora-torture-cop-kicked-out-of-force/.

20. "Every Guyanese Needs to Speak Out to End Police Brutality," *Stabroek News*,
January 30, 2014, http://www.pressreader.com/guyana/stabroek-news/20140130
/281556583703050.

## Chapter 2. Who Are the Torture Doctors?

1. Cari Romm, "Rethinking One of Psychology's Most Infamous Experiments,"
*Atlantic*, January 28, 1915, https://www.theatlantic.com/health/archive/2015/01
/rethinking-one-of-psychologys-most-infamous-experiments/384913/.

2. Ethan B. Ludmir, Muhammad Ali Elahi, and Barak D. Richman, "The Physician
as Dictator," *Lancet* 390, no. 10099 (September 2017): 1023, https://doi.org/10
.1016/s0140–6736(17)32147–5.

3. Prosecutor v. Milomir Stakić, IT-97–24-T, Judgment (International Criminal Tribunal for the Former Yugoslavia, 2003).

4. Julian Borger and Owen Bowcott, "Radovan Karadžić Sentenced to 40 Years for Srebrenica Genocide," *Guardian*, March 24, 2016, https://www.theguardian.com/world/2016/mar/24/radovan-karadzic-criminally-responsible-for-genocide-at-srebenica.

5. Trial International, "Milan Kovacevic," December 23, 2009, last modified October 16, 2016, https://trialinternational.org/latest-post/milan-kovacevic/.

6. Prosecutor v. Blagoje Simić et al., IT-95–9-T, Judgment (International Criminal Tribunal for the Former Yugoslavia, 2003).

7. Prosecutor v. Blagoje Simić, IT-95–9-ES, Decision of President on Early Release of Blagoje Simić (International Criminal Tribunal for the Former Yugoslavia, 2011).

8. Prosecutor v. Elizaphan et al., ICTR-96–10 and ICTR-96–17-T, Judgment and Sentence (International Criminal Tribunal for Rwanda, 2003).

9. Prosecutor v. Clement Kayishema et al., ICTR-96–1-T, Sentence (International Criminal Tribunal for Rwanda, 1999).

10. Prosecutor v. Niyitegeka, ITCR-96–14-T, Judgment and Sentence (International Criminal Tribunal for Rwanda, 2003).

11. Lucia Villela, "The Chalice of Silence and the Case That Refuses to Go Away," *Psychoanalytic Review* 92, no. 6 (December 2005): 807–28, https://doi.org/10.1521/prev.2005.92.6.807.

12. Robert Proctor, *Racial Hygiene: Medicine under the Nazis* (Cambridge, MA: Harvard University Press, 2002), 62–94.

13. Vivien Spitz, *Doctors from Hell: The Horrific Account of Nazi Experiments on Humans* (Boulder, CO: Sentient Publications, 2005), 190.

14. Helena B. Vianna, "O Real Da Ética" [The reality of ethics], lecture, Tours, France, October 17, 1998, http://egp.dreamhosters.com/EGP/89-o_real_da_etica.shtml; Amílcar Lobo, *A Hora do Lobo e a Hora do Carneiro* [The hour of the wolf and the hour of the sheep], quoted by H. V. Besserman, "O Real da Ética," *Discursividad Analítica*, August 17, 1998, https://discursividadanalitica.com/documentos-para-la-lectura-la-etificacion-del-psicoanalisis-de-jean-allouch/.

15. Eric Stover, ed., *The Open Secret: Torture and the Medical Profession in Chile* (Washington, DC: American Association for the Advancement of Science, 1987), 67.

16. John Duckitt et al., "The Psychological Basis of Ideology and Prejudice: Testing a Dual Process Model," *Journal of Personality and Social Psychology* 83, no. 1 (July 2002): 75–93, https://doi.org/10.1037//0022–3514.83.1.75.

17. Alfredo Jadresic, "Doctors and Torture: An Experience as a Prisoner," *Journal of Medical Ethics* 6, no. 3 (September 1980): 124–27, https://doi.org/10.1136/jme.6.3.124.

18. Jun Hongo, "Vivisectionist Recalls His Day of Reckoning," *Japan Times*, October 24, 2007, http://www.japantimes.co.jp/news/2007/10/24/reference/special-presentations/vivisectionist-recalls-his-day-of-reckoning/.

19. Cristina Grillo, "Minha História: Meu marido não foi um torturador" [My story: My husband was not a torturer], *Folha de Sao Paulo*, June 16, 2013, http://www1.folha.uol.com.br/poder/2013/06/1295643-minha-historia-meu-marido-nao-foi-um-torturador.shtml.

20. Nicholas Kulish and Souad Mekhennet, *The Eternal Nazi: From Mauthausen to Cairo, the Relentless Pursuit of SS Doctor Aribert Heim* (New York: Doubleday, 2014).
21. Sidney Bloch and Peter Reddaway, *Russia's Political Hospitals: The Abuse of Psychiatry in the Soviet Union* (London: Victor Gollancz, 1977), 329.
22. Stover and Nightingale, *Breaking of Bodies and Minds*, 150.
23. Lawrence C. James, *Fixing Hell: An Army Psychologist Confronts Abu Ghraib* (New York: Grand Central, 2008), 180–81.
24. Toby Harnden, "James Mitchell, CIA's 'Torture Teacher' Hits Back," *Real Clear Politics*, December 16, 2014, https://www.realclearpolitics.com/articles/2014/12/16/james_mitchell_cias_torture_teacher_hits_back_124968-3.html.
25. Emily Gosden, "Saddam Hussein's 'Torture Doctor' Worked in NHS," *Telegraph*, July 2, 2011, https://www.telegraph.co.uk/news/uknews/immigration/8612273/Saddam-Husseins-torture-doctor-worked-in-NHS-hospital.html.
26. Chris Bateman, "Bio-ethics Vigilance Vital: Medical and Legal Doyens," *South African Medical Journal* 99, no. 5 (May 2009): 298–99, http://www.scielo.org.za/scielo.php?pid=S0256-95742009000500010&script=sci_arttext.
27. Cecilia Devanna, "No sé para que las cuidamos tanto si después las tiramos al río" [I do not know why we take care of them so much if we later throw them into the river], Infojus Noticias, June 10, 2014, http://www.infojusnoticias.gov.ar/nacionales/no-se-para-que-las-cuidamos-tanto-si-despues-las-tiramos-al-rio-5950.html.
28. Stanley Milgram, *Obedience to Authority: An Experimental View* (New York: Harper Perennial, 2009); Jerry M. Burger, "Replicating Milgram: Would People Still Obey Today?," *American Psychology* 64, no. 1 (January 2009): 1–11, https://doi.org/10.1037/a0010932.
29. V. Lee Hamilton and Herbert C. Kelman, *Crimes of Obedience: Toward a Social Psychology of Authority and Responsibility* (New Haven, CT: Yale University Press, 1990).
30. Michael J. Osofsky, Albert Bandura, and Philip G. Zimbardo, "The Role of Moral Disengagement in the Execution Process," *Law and Human Behavior* 29, no. 4 (August 2005): 371–93, https://doi.org/10.1007/s10979-005-4930-1.
31. Erving Goffman, *Asylums: Essays on the Social Situation of Mental Patients and Other Inmates* (Harmondsworth, UK: Penguin, 1968); Jerrold M. Post and Lara K. Panis, "Crimes of Obedience: 'Groupthink' at Abu Ghraib," *International Journal of Group Psychotherapy* 61, no. 1 (January 2011): 48–66, https://doi.org/10.1521/ijgp.2011.61.1.48.
32. Janice T. Gibson and Mika Haritos-Farouros, "The Education of a Torturer," *Psychology Today* 20, no. 11 (November 1986): 50–52, 56–58, https://doi.org/10.1037/e400772009-004; Jessica Wolfendale, *Torture and the Military Profession* (New York: Palgrave Macmillan, 2007).
33. Robert J. Lifton, *The Nazi Doctors: Medical Killing and the Psychology of Genocide* (New York: Basic Books, 1986), 418–65; Robert J. Lifton, *Home from the War* (New York: Other Press, 1973), 41–71.
34. Alexander Mitscherlich and Fred Mielke, *Doctors of Infamy*, trans. Heinz Norden (New York: Henry Schuman, 1949), 417–65.

35. Peter Vesti and Neils J. Lavik, "Torture and the Medical Profession: A Review," *Journal of Medical Ethics* S17 (December 1, 1991): 4–8, https://doi.org/10.1136/jme.17.suppl.4.
36. Mitscherlich and Mielke, *Doctors of Infamy*, 322.
37. Philip Zimbardo, *The Lucifer Effect: Understanding How Good People Turn Evil* (New York: Random House, 2007), 220.
38. Jacobo Timerman, *Prisoner without a Name, Cell without a Number* (New York: Knopf, 1981), 54.
39. Gosden, "Saddam Hussein's 'Torture Doctor.'"
40. Robert van Voren, "Political Abuse of Psychiatry—An Historical Overview," *Schizophrenia Bulletin* 36, no. 1 (January 2010): 33–35, https://doi.org/10.1093/schbul/sbp119.
41. Jadresic, "Doctors and Torture," 124–27.
42. Spitz, *Doctors from Hell*, 258–64; Sheldon H. Harris, *Factories of Death: Japanese Biological Warfare, 1932–1945, and the American Cover Up*, 2nd ed. (New York: Routledge, 2002).
43. Spitz, *Doctors from Hell*, 261.
44. David A. Hackett, trans. and ed., *The Buchenwald Report* (Boulder, CO: Westview Press, 1995), 79.
45. Harris, *Factories of Death*, 56.
46. Darius M. Rejali, *Torture and Democracy* (Princeton, NJ: Princeton University Press, 2007), 243–47, 420–25.
47. Villela, "Chalice of Silence," 807–28.
48. Fernanda Canofre, "5 Accounts from Female Political Prisoners That Recall the Horrific Torture under Brazil's Military Dictatorship," trans. Liam Anderson, *Global Voices*, June 28, 2016, https://globalvoices.org/2016/06/28/5-accounts-from-female-political-prisoners-that-recall-the-horrific-torture-under-brazils-military-dictatorship/.
49. Leo Alexander, "Medical Science under Dictatorship," *New England Journal of Medicine* 241, no. 2 (July 14, 1949): 39–47, https://doi.org/10.1056/NEJM194907142410201.
50. Knud Smidt-Nielson, "The Participation of Health Professionals in Torture," *Torture* 8 (1998): 91–94.
51. Amnesty International and Medical Association of Chile, *Participation of Physicians in Torture*, AMR 22/36/86, 1986, http://link.library.missouri.edu/portal/Chile-human-rights-in-Chile—the-role-of-the/z59qDZHLSsk/.
52. Jadresic, "Doctors and Torture," 124–27.
53. Lifton, *Nazi Doctors*, 214–55.
54. John Heminway, *In Full Flight: A Story of Africa and Atonement* (New York: Knopf, 2018).
55. Spitz, *Doctors from Hell*, 66.
56. Claus A. Pierach, "Give Me a Break: Gerhard Küntscher and His Nail," *Perspectives in Biology and Medicine* 57, no. 3 (Summer 2014): 361–73, https://dx.doi.org/10.1353/pbm.2014.0021.

57. Amnesty International and the Medical Association of Chile, *Participation of Physicians in Torture*, 27.

58. John S. Yudkin, "The Israeli Medical Association and Doctors' Complicity in Torture," *British Medical Journal* 339 (October 7, 2009): b4078, https://doi.org/10.1136/bmj.b4078.

59. Chen Reis et al., "Physician Participation in Human Rights Abuses in Southern Iraq," *JAMA* 291, no. 12 (March 2004): 1480–86, https://doi.org/10.1001/jama.291.12.1480; Samir Johna, "Anatomija zločina: Liječnici za vrijeme represivnoga režima Saddama Husseina" [The anatomy of crime: Physicians under the oppressive regime of Saddam Hussein], *Acta Medico—Storica Adriatica* 7, no. 2 (2009): 303–8, https://zdoc.site/physicians-under-the-oppressive-regime-of-saddam-hussein.html.

60. Mitscherlich and Mielke, *Doctors of Infamy*, xxxii.

61. Spitz, *Doctors from Hell*, 50; Proctor, *Racial Hygiene*, 66.

62. *World Medical Association Bulletin* 1, no. 1 (1949): 3–14; Amnesty International and the Medical Association of Chile, *Participation of Physicians in Torture*, 27.

63. "Alleged Police Torture: PHC Cancels Doctor's Transfer Orders," *Express Tribune*, October 11, 2012, http://tribune.com.pk/story/449889/alleged-police-torture-phc-cancels-doctors-transfer-orders/.

64. Grillo, "Minha História."

65. Jesper Sonntag, "Doctors' Involvement in Torture," *Torture* 18, no. 3 (February 2008): 161–75, https://pdfs.semanticscholar.org/91da/3f051f97260c0373462eba00da0c616c33b8.pdf; Physicians for Human Rights (PHR), *Dual Loyalty and Human Rights in Health Professional Practice: Proposed Guidelines and Institutional Mechanisms*, March 2003, http://physiciansforhumanrights.org/library/reports/dual-loyalty-and-human-rights-2003.html; Jerome A. Singh, "American Physicians and Dual Loyalty Obligations in the 'War on Terror,'" *BMC Medical Ethics* 4, no. 4 (August 1, 2003), https://doi.org/10.1186/1472-6939-4-4.

## Chapter 3. What Is Torture?

1. UN General Assembly, Resolution 39/46, Convention against Torture and Other Cruel, Inhuman or Degrading Treatment or Punishment, A/RES/39/46 (December 10, 1984), http://www.ohchr.org/EN/ProfessionalInterest/Pages/CAT.aspx.

2. World Medical Association (WMA), *Guidelines for Physicians concerning Torture and Other Cruel, Inhuman or Degrading Treatment or Punishment in Relation to Detention and Imprisonment (Declaration of Tokyo)*, October 1975, revised October 2016, https://www.wma.net/policies-post/wma-declaration-of-tokyo-guidelines-for-physicians-concerning-torture-and-other-cruel-inhuman-or-degrading-treatment-or-punishment-in-relation-to-detention-and-imprisonment/.

3. UN General Assembly, Resolution 37/194, Principles of Medical Ethics Relevant to the Role of Health Personnel, particularly Physicians, in the Protection of Prisoners and Detainees against Torture and Other Cruel, Inhuman or Degrading Treatment or Punishment, A/RES/37/194 (December 18, 1982), http://www

.ohchr.org/EN/ProfessionalInterest/Pages/MedicalEthics.aspx, http://www.un.org/documents/ga/res/37/a37r194.htm.

4. Association for Prevention of Torture, https://www.apt.ch/en/who-we-are/.

5. Elie Wiesel, "Without Conscience," *New England Journal of Medicine* 352 (2005): 1511–13.

6. Darius M. Rejali, *Torture and Modernity: Self, Society and State in Modern Iran* (Boulder, CO: Westview Press, 1994), 13.

7. Rejali, *Torture and Democracy*, 163–70.

8. Malise Ruthven, *Torture: The Grand Conspiracy* (London: Weidenfeld and Nicolson, 1978), 25–31, 282–83.

9. Jay Bybee, *Standards for Conduct for Interrogation under 18 U.S.C. 2340–2340A* (Washington, DC: US Department of Justice Office of Legal Counsel, August 1, 2002), https://www.justice.gov/olc/file/886061/download.

10. Nigel S. Rodley, "The Definition(s) of Torture in International Law," *Current Legal Problems* 55, no. 1 (2002): 467–93, https://doi.org/10.1093/clp/55.1.467.

11. UN High Commissioner for Refugees, *Protecting Refugees: Questions and Answers*, February 1, 2002, http://www.unhcr.org/afr/publications/brochures/3b779dfe2/protecting-refugees-questions-answers.html.

12. "Australia: Appalling Abuse, Neglect of Refugees on Nauru," Human Rights Watch, August 2016, https://www.hrw.org/news/2016/08/02/australia-appalling-abuse-neglect-refugees-nauru; and Amnesty International, *Australia's Regime of Cruelty Has Turned Nauru into an Open-Air Prison*, ASA 12/4934/2016, 2016, https://www.amnesty.org.au/island-of-despair-nauru-refugee-report-2016/.

13. UN Human Rights Council, Report of the Special Rapporteur on Torture and Other Cruel, Inhuman or Degrading Treatment or Punishment, A/HRC/28/68/Add.1 (March 6, 2015), 7–9, https://static.guim.co.uk/ni/1425873116713/Mendez-report.pdf; Amnesty International, *Australia: Island of Despair: Australia's 'Processing' of Refugees on Nauru*, ASA 12/4934/2016, October 17, 2016, https://www.amnesty.org/en/documents/asa12/4934/2016/en/; and Australia Lawyers for Human Rights, *Joint NGO Report on Australia to the UN Committee against Torture*, November 12, 2014, https://alhr.org.au/%EF%BF%BC%EF%BF%BC%EF%BF%BCjoint-ngo-report-australia-un-committee-torture/.

14. Mary Lowth, "Australia and the Nauru Files: Doctors Fighting for the Human Rights of Asylum Seekers," *British Journal of General Practice* 67, no. 663 (2017): 465–66, https://doi.org/10.3399/bjgp17X692861; Elizabeth Schumacher, "Australia Doctors Refuse to Discharge Refugee Baby for Detention on Nauru," *Deutche Welle*, February 13, 2016, https://www.dw.com/en/australia-doctors-refuse-to-discharge-refugee-baby-for-detention-on-nauru/a-19046995; and Ben Doherty and Saba Vasefi, "Asylum Seeker Boy on Nauru Pleads for Medical Help for His Mother," *Guardian*, April 25, 2018, https://www.theguardian.com/australia-news/2018/apr/25/asylum-seeker-boy-on-nauru-pleads-for-medical-help-for-his-mother.

15. Royal Australian and New Zealand College of Psychiatrists, *Position Statement 46: The Provision of Mental Health Services for Asylum Seekers and Refugees*, September

2017, https://docs.wixstatic.com/ugd/b05174_06186919833648118dd209fb70
d1e0f1.pdf.

16. Doctors for Refugees, https://www.doctors4refugees.org/new-form-test-page.

17. Ben Doherty, "Nauru Doctor Wins Global Free Speech Award for Speaking Out
on Offshore Immigration," *Guardian*, January 16, 2019, https://www.theguardian
.com/australia-news/2019/jan/17/nauru-doctor-wins-global-free-speech-award
-for-speaking-out-on-offshore-immigration; and Nick Martin, "As Doctors
Working on Nauru, We Thought We Were Helping. Now I Know We Were Not,"
*Guardian*, October 11, 2018, https://www.theguardian.com/commentisfree/2018
/oct/12/as-doctors-working-on-nauru-we-thought-we-were-helping-now-i-know
-we-were-not.

18. Alex McDonald, "Save the Children Offices on Nauru Raided for Second Time
by Police," *ABC News* (Australia), October 22, 2015, http://www.abc.net.au
/news/2015-10-22/save-the-children-offices-on-nauru-raided-for-second-time
/6876444.

19. Parliament of Australia, Australian Border Force Bill, Parliament no. 44 (2015),
https://www.aph.gov.au/Parliamentary_Business/Bills_Legislation/Bills_Search
_Results/Result?bId=r5408.

20. David Berger and Steven H. Miles, "Should Doctors Boycott Working in Australia's Immigration Detention Centres?," *British Medical Journal* 352 (March
2016): 1600.

21. Aaron Hegarty, "Timeline: Immigrant Children Separated from Families at the
Border," *USA Today*, June 27, 2017, https://www.usatoday.com/story/news/2018
/06/27/immigrant-children-family-separation-border-timeline/734014002/.

22. Miriam Jordan, "Family Separation May Have Hit Thousands More Migrant
Children than Reported," *New York Times*, January 17, 2019, https://www.nytimes
.com/2019/01/17/us/family-separation-trump-administration-migrants.html.

23. Miriam Jordan, "Trump Administration Says It Needs More Time to Reunite
Migrant Families," *New York Times*, July 6, 2018, https://www.nytimes.com/2018
/07/06/us/migrant-children-court-families.html.

24. "Release Migrant Children from Detention and Stop Using Them to Deter Irregular Migration," UN Office of the High Commissioner for Human Rights, June
22, 2018, https://ohchr.org/EN/NewsEvents/Pages/DisplayNews.aspx?NewsID=
23245&LangID=E.

25. Ingrid Eagley, Steven Shafer, and Jana Whalley, "Detaining Families: A Study
of Asylum Adjudication in Family Detention," *California Law Review* 106
(2018): 785–830, https://doi.org/10.15779/Z38WH2DF26.

26. American Academy of Pediatrics, "Statement Opposing Separation of Children and Parents at the Border," news release, May 8, 2018, https://www
.aap.org/en-us/about-the-aap/aap-press-room/Pages/StatementOpposing
SeparationofChildrenandParents.aspx; American College of Physicians, "ACP
Objects to Separation of Children from Their Parents at Border," news
release, May 30, 2018, https://www.acponline.org/acp-newsroom/acp-objects
-to-separation-of-children-from-their-parents-at-border; American Psychiatric

Association, "Statement Opposing Separation of Children from Parents at the Border," news release, May 30, 2018, https://www.psychiatry.org/newsroom/news -releases/apa-statement-opposing-separation-of-children-from-parents-at-the -border; and American Medical Association, "Doctors Oppose Policy That Splits Kids from Caregivers at Border," news release, June 13, 2018, https://wire.ama -assn.org/ama-news/doctors-oppose-policy-splits-kids-caregivers-border.

27. Blake Ellis, Melanie Hicken, and Bob Ortega, "Handcuffs, Assaults, and Drugs Called 'Vitamins': Children Allege Grave Abuse at Migrant Detention Facilities," CNN, June 21, 2018, https://www.cnn.com/2018/06/21/us/undocumented -migrant-children-detention-facilities-abuse-invs/index.html; Matt Smith and Aura Bogado, "Immigrant Children Forcibly Injected with Drugs at Texas Shelter, Lawsuit Claims," *Texas Tribune*, June 20, 2018, https://www.texastribune .org/2018/06/20/immigrant-children-forcibly-injected-drugs-lawsuit-claims/; Jan C. Costello and Elizabeth J. Jameson, "Legal and Ethical Duties of Health Care Professionals to Incarcerated Children," *Journal of Legal Medicine* 8, no. 2 (1987): 191–263, https://doi.org/10.1080/01947648709513498; Samantha Schmidt, "Trump Administration Must Stop Giving Psychotropic Drugs to Migrant Children without Consent, Judge Rules," *Washington Post*, July 31, 2018, https://www.washingtonpost.com/news/morning-mix/wp/2018/07/31/trump -administration-must-seek-consent-before-giving-drugs-to-migrant-children -judge-rules; and Scott J. Schweikart, "April 2018 Flores Settlement Suit Challenges Unlawful Administration of Psychotropic Medication to Immigrant Children," *AMA Journal of Ethics* 21, no. 1 (2019): 67–72, https://doi.org/10.1001 /amajethics.2019.67.

28. UN General Assembly, Resolution 44/25, Convention on the Rights of the Child, A/RES/44/25 (September 2, 1990), art. 3, 5, 8, 9, 10, 16, 22, and 37, https://www .ohchr.org/en/professionalinterest/pages/crc.aspx.

29. Adam Hochschild, *Bury the Chains: Prophets and Rebels in the Fight to Free an Empire's Slaves* (Boston: Mariner Books, 2006), 11.

30. Cesare Bonesana di Beccaria, "Of Torture," in *An Essay on Crimes and Punishments (1760)* (Albany, NY: W. C. Little, 1872), http://www.constitution.org/cb /crim_pun16.htm.

31. Steven Pinker, *The Better Angels of Our Nature: Why Violence Has Declined* (New York: Penguin Books, 2012), 149.

32. Tania Nicole Masmas et al., "Asylum Seekers in Denmark—A Study of Health Status and Grade of Traumatization of Newly Arrived Asylum Seekers," *Torture* 18, no. 2 (February 2008): 77–86, https://www.researchgate.net/publication /24204264_Asylum_seekers_in_Denmark—a_study_of_health_status_and_grade _of_traumatization_of_newly_arrived_asylum_seekers, 77–86; James Sanders, Melissa W. Schuman, and Anne M. Marbella, "The Epidemiology of Torture: A Case Series of 58 Survivors of Torture," *Forensic Science International* 189, nos. 1–3 (August 2009): 1–7, https://doi.org/10.1016/j.forsciint.2009.03.026; Edward Domovitch et al., "Human Torture: Description and Sequelae of 104 Cases," *Canadian Family Physician* 30 (April 1984): 827–30; Steven H. Miles and Rosa E. Garcia-Peltoniemi, "Torture Survivors: What to Ask, How to Document," *Journal*

*of Family Practice* 61, no. 4 (April 2012): 1–5, https://www.cvt.org/sites/default /files/downloads/Torture%20Survivors%20What%20to%20ask%2C%20how %20to%20document_Journal%20of%20Family%20Practice_April2012.pdf; and Joshua B. Hooberman et al., "Classifying the Torture Experiences of Refugees Living in the United States," *Journal of InterpersonalViolence* 22, no. 1 (2007): 108–23, https://doi.org/10.1177/0886260506294999.

33. Kirstine Amris, Soren Torp-Pedersen, and Ole V. Rasmussen, "Long-Term Consequences of Falanga Torture—What Do We Know and What Do We Need to Know?," *Torture* 19, no. 1 (2009): 33–40, https://irct.org/assets/uploads/1018 _8185_2009–1_33–40.pdf; Erik Edston, "The Epidemiology of Falanga: Incidence among Swedish Asylum Seekers," *Torture* 19, no. 1 (2009): 27–32, https:// irct.org/assets/uploads/1018_8185_2009–1_28–32.pdf.

34. Mladen Loncar, Neven Henigsberg, and Pero Hrabac, "Mental Health Consequences in Men Exposed to Sexual Abuse during the War in Croatia and Bosnia," *Journal of InterpersonalViolence* 25, no. 2 (2009): 191–203, https://doi.org/10.1177 /0886260509334288.

35. Richard F. Mollica et al., "Brain Structural Abnormalities and Mental Health Sequelae in South Vietnamese Ex-Political Detainees Who Survived Traumatic Head Injury andTorture," *Archives of General Psychiatry* 66, no. 11 (2009): 1221–32, https://doi.org/10.1001/archgenpsychiatry.2009.127.

36. Alejandro Moreno and Michael A. Grodin, "Torture and Its Neurological Sequelae," *Spinal Cord* 40, no. 5 (2002): 213–23, https://doi.org/10.1038/sj.sc .3101284; Dorte R. Olsen et al., "Prevalent Musculoskeletal Pain as a Correlate of Previous Exposure to Torture," *Scandinavian Journal of Public Health* 34, no. 5 (2006): 496–503, https://doi.org/10.1080/14034940600554677.

37. Erik Edston, "The Epidemiology of Falanga," *Torture* 19 (2009): 27–32, https:// www.researchgate.net/publication/26262050_The_epidemiology_of_falanga— incidence_among_Swedish_asylum_seekers; Pauline Oosterhoff, Prisca Zwanikken, and Evert Ketting, "Sexual Torture of Men in Croatia and Other Conflict Situations: An Open Secret," *Reproductive Health Matters* 12, no. 23 (2004): 68–77, https://doi.org/10.1016/s0968–8080(04)23115–9.

38. Cheryl L. Robertson et al., "Somali and Oromo Refugee Women: Trauma and Associated Factors," *Journal of Advanced Nursing* 56 (2006): 577–87, https://doi .org/10.1111/j.1365–2648.2006.04057.x; Miles and Garcia-Peltoniemi, "Torture Survivors," 1–5.

39. Allen Keller et al., "Traumatic Experiences and Psychological Distress in an Urban Refugee Population Seeking Treatment Services," *Journal of Nervous and Mental Disease* 194, no. 3 (2006): 188–94, https://doi.org/10.1097/01.nmd .0000202494.75723.83; Inge Lunde and Jorgen Ortmann, "Prevalence and Sequelae of SexualTorture," *Lancet* 336, no. 8710 (1990): 289–91, https://doi.org /10.1016/0140–6736(90)91814-q.

40. Metin Başoğlu, Maria Livanou, and Cvetana Crnobarić, "Torture vs Other Cruel, Inhuman, and Degrading Treatment," *Archives of General Psychiatry* 64, no. 3 (2007): 277–85, https://doi.org/10.1001/archpsyc.64.3.277; Metin Başoğlu et al., "Psychiatric and Cognitive Effects of War in Former Yugoslavia: Association of

Lack of Redress for Trauma and Posttraumatic Stress Reactions," *JAMA* 294, no. 5 (August 2005): 580–90, https://doi.org/10.1001/jama.294.5.580; Mark Van Ommeren et al., "Psychiatric Disorders among Tortured Bhutanese Refugees in Nepal," *Archives of General Psychiatry* 58, no. 5 (2001): 475–82, https://doi.org /10.1001/archpsyc.58.5.475; Andrew Rasmussen et al., "The Effects of Torture-Related Injuries on Long-Term Psychological Distress in a Punjabi Sikh Sample," *Journal of Abnormal Psychology* 116, no. 4 (2007): 734–40, https://doi.org/10.1037 /0021–843x.116.4.734; Olsen et al., "Prevalent Musculoskeletal Pain," 496–503; Dorte R. Olsen et al., "Prevalent Pain and Pain Level among Torture Survivors: A Follow-Up Study," *Danish Medical Bulletin* 53, no. 2 (May 2006): 210–14; and Metin Başoğlu, "A Multivariate Contextual Analysis of Torture and Cruel, Inhuman, and Degrading Treatments: Implications for an Evidence-Based Definition of Torture," *American Journal of Orthopsychiatry* 79, no. 2 (2009): 135–45, https:// doi.org/10.1037/a0015681.

41. Masmas et al., "Asylum Seekers in Denmark," 77–86; and Richard F. Mollica, "Surviving Torture," *New England Journal of Medicine* 351 (July 2004): 5–7, https://doi.org/10.1056/NEJMp048141.

42. Andrew Steptoe and Lena Brydon, "Emotional Triggering of Cardiac Events," *Neuroscience and Biobehavioral Reviews* 33, no. 2 (February 2009): 63–70, https:// doi.org/10.1016/j.neubiorev.2008.04.010.

43. Jessica M. Carlsson et al., "Mental Health and Health-Related Quality of Life: A 10-Year Follow-Up of Tortured Refugees," *Journal of Nervous and Mental Disease* 194, no. 10 (2006): 725–31, https://doi.org/10.1097/01.nmd.0000243079 .52138.b7; Başoğlu, Livanou, and Crnobarić, "Torture vs Other," 277–85; Stuart W. Turner and Caroline Gorst-Unsworth, "Psychological Sequelae of Torture," in *International Handbook of Traumatic Stress Syndromes*, ed. John P. Beverly and Raphael Wilson (New York: Plenum Press, 1993), 703–13.

44. Richard D. Blackwell, "Disruption and Reconstitution of Family, Network, and Community Systems following Torture, Organized Violence, and Exile," in Beverly and Wilson, *International Handbook*, 733–41.

45. Jean M. Arrigo, "A Utilitarian Argument against Torture Interrogation of Terrorists," *Science and Engineering Ethics* 10, no. 3 (2004): 543–72, https://doi.org/10 .1007/s11948-004-0011-y.

46. Central Intelligence Agency (CIA) v. Sims, 471 U.S. 159 (1985).

47. CIA, *KUBARK Counterintelligence Interrogation Manual*, July 1963, https:// nsarchive2.gwu.edu/nsaebb/nsaebb27/docs/doc01.pdf.

48. CIA, *Human Resource Exploitation Manual*, 1983, https://archive.org/details/CIA _Human_Resource_Exploitation_Manual/page/n9.

49. Headquarters, US Department of the Army, *FM 34–52 Intelligence Interrogation*, May 1987, https://www.loc.gov/rr/frd/Military_Law/pdf/intel_interrogation_may -1987.pdf.

50. CIA, *Brainwashing from a Psychological Viewpoint*, 1956, 1–92, https://www.cia.gov /library/readingroom/docs/CIA-RDP65–00756R000400050004–9.pdf.

51. Julius Segal, "Correlates of Collaboration and Resistance Behavior among U.S. Army POWs in Korea," *Journal of Social Issues* 13, no. 3 (1957): 31–40, https:// doi.org/10.1111/j.1540–4560.1957.tb02268.x.

52. US Department of Defense, *Working Group Report on Detainee Interrogations in the Global War on Terrorism*, April 4, 2003, 52, http://www2.gwu.edu/~nsarchiv/nsaebb/nsaebb127/03.04.04.pdf.

53. Russell Swenson, ed., *Educing Information: Interrogation: Science and Art: Foundations for the Future: Intelligence Science Board Phase 1 Report* (Washington, DC: National Defense Intelligence College Press, 2006), 58.

54. CIA, *KUBARK*.

55. Chris Mackey and Greg Miller, *The Interrogators: Inside the Secret War against Al Qaeda* (New York: Little, Brown, 2004).

56. CIA, *Human Resource Exploitation Manual*, 1983, https://archive.org/details/CIAHumanResourceExploitationManual.

57. Reza Afshari, "Tortured Confessions: Prisons and Public Recantations in Modern Iran," *Human Rights Quarterly* 24, no. 1 (2002): 290–97, https://doi.org/10.1353/hrq.2002.0001; Miles, *Oath Betrayed*, 16–17, 44.

58. Rex A. Hudson, *The Sociology and Psychology of Terrorism: Who Becomes a Terrorist and Why?* (Washington, DC: Federal Research Division, Library of Congress, 1999), http://www.loc.gov/rr/frd/pdf-files/Soc_Psych_of_Terrorism.pdf.

59. Paul Aussaresses, *The Battle of the Casbah: Terrorism and Counter-Terrorism in Algeria, 1955–1957* (New York: Enigma Books, 2010).

60. Fareed Zakaria, "Pssst . . . Nobody Loves a Torturer," *Newsweek*, November 14, 2005.

61. Colin Powell, "Draft Decision Memorandum for the President on the Applicability of the Geneva Convention to the Conflict in Afghanistan," in *The Torture Papers: The Road to Abu Ghraib*, ed. Karen J. Greenberg and Joshua Dratel (Cambridge: Cambridge University Press, 2005), 122–25; William Howard Taft IV, "Comments on Your Paper on the Geneva Convention," February 2, 2002, in Greenberg and Dratel, *Torture Papers*, 129–33; US Department of State, Bureau of Democracy, Human Rights, and Labor, *Country Reports on Human Rights Practices: China (Includes Tibet, Hong Kong, and Macau)*, 2005, https://www.state.gov/j/drl/rls/hrrpt/2004/41640.htm.

62. "Working Group Report on Detainee Interrogations in the Global War on Terrorism" (April 2003), in Greenfield and Dratel, *Torture Papers*, 335–36, 346.

63. Dana Priest, "CIA Puts Harsh Tactics on Hold," *Washington Post*, June 27, 2004.

64. "Working Group Report on Detainee Interrogations."

65. Lifton, *Home from the War*, 41–71.

66. Rachel M. MacNair, "Perpetration-Induced Traumatic Stress in Combat Veterans," *Peace and Conflict: Journal of Peace Psychology* 8, no. 1 (2002): 63–67, https://doi.org/10.1207/s15327949pac0801_6; Lifton, *Home from the War*, 41–71; and Melinda Dee, "Effect of Torture on the Torturer," *GlobalJusticeBlog.com*, November 27, 2017, http://www.law.utah.edu/effect-of-torture-on-the-torturer/#_ftnref39.

67. Fyodor Dostoevsky, *The Brothers Karamazov*, trans. Constance Garnett (New York: Barnes and Nobles Classics, 1912), 227.

68. Charles A. Pfaff, "Toward an Ethics of Detention and Interrogation: Consent and Limits," *Philosophy and Public Policy Quarterly* 25, no. 3 (2005): 18–21, https://journals.gmu.edu/PPPQ/article/download/181/122; and Fritz Allhoff, "Terrorism

and Torture," *International Journal of Applied Philosophy* 17, no. 1 (2003): 121–34, https://doi.org/10.5840/ijap200317113.

69. Alan Dershowitz, "Tortured Reasoning," in *Torture: A Collection,* ed. Sanford Levinson (New York: Oxford University Press, 2004), 257–80.

70. Association for the Prevention of Torture, *Defusing the Ticking Bomb Scenario: Why We Must Say No to Torture, Always,* 2007, https://www.apt.ch/c.

## Chapter 4. What Is a Torture Doctor?

1. Jesper Sonntag, "Doctors' Involvement in Torture," *Torture* 18, no. 3 (2008): 161–75.

2. WMA, *Declaration of Tokyo—Guidelines for Medical Doctors concerning Torture and Other Cruel, Inhuman or Degrading Treatment or Punishment in Relation to Detention and Imprisonment,* October 1975, http://www.cirp.org/library/ethics/tokyo/.

3. UN General Assembly, Resolution 37/194.

4. Rejali, *Torture and Democracy,* 427–30.

5. Michael W. Lewis, "A Dark Descent into Reality: Making the Case for an Objective Definition of Torture," *Washington and Lee Law Review* 67, no. 1 (January 2010): 77–136.

6. Amnesty International, *Involvement of Medical Personnel in Abuses against Detainees and Prisoners (Revised and Updated),* ACT 75/08/90, November 1990, http://www.amnesty.org/ar/library/asset/ACT75/008/1990/en/a5ddbc58-ee66–11dd-96f1–9fdd7e6f4873/act750081990en.pdf; and Amnesty International, *Declaration on the Role of Health Professionals in the Exposure of Torture and Ill-Treatment,* March 31, 1996, https://www.amnesty.org/download/Documents/172000/pol300 021996en.pdf00021996en.pdf.

7. Rejali, *Torture and Democracy,* 8–16.

## Chapter 5. Judging the Nazi Doctors

1. Franklin Roosevelt, Winston Churchill, and Joseph Stalin, *Moscow Declaration on Atrocities,* November 1, 1943, https://www.cvce.eu/content/publication/2004/2/12/699fc03f-19a1–47f0-aec0–73220489efcd/publishable_en.pdf.

2. US Holocaust Memorial Museum, *Holocaust Encyclopedia,* s.v. "Ohrdruf," accessed June 8, 2019, https://www.ushmm.org/wlc/en/article.php?ModuleId= 10006131.

3. Proctor, *Racial Hygiene*; Götz Aly, Peter Chroust, and Christian Pross, *Cleansing the Fatherland: Nazi Medicine and Racial Hygiene,* trans. Belinda Cooper (Baltimore: Johns Hopkins University Press, 1994); Lifton, *Nazi Doctors*; and Benno Müller-Hill, *Murderous Science: Elimination by Scientific Selection of Jews, Gypsies, and Others, Germany, 1933–1945,* trans. George R. Fraser (New York: Oxford University Press, 1988).

4. William E. Seidelman, "An Inquiry into the Spiritual Death of Dr. Hippocrates," *Harefuah* 120, no. 11 (June 2, 1991): 677–82, https://www.ncbi.nlm.nih.gov /pubmed/1937221.

5. Paul J. Weindling, *John W. Thompson: Psychiatrist in the Shadow of the Holocaust* (Rochester, NY: University of Rochester Press, 2010).

6. Felix Lancashire, "The British Advisory Committee for Medical War Crimes," *Royal College of Physicians Blog*, January 26, 2018, https://history .rcplondon.ac.uk/blog/these-grim-documents-physicians-responses-nazi -medical-war-crimes.

7. Ann Tusa and John Tusa, *The Nuremberg Trial* (New York: Atheneum Publishers, 1984); Whitney R. Harris, *Tyranny on Trial: The Trial of the Major War Criminals at the End of World War II at Nuremberg, Germany, 1945–1946* (Dallas: Southern Methodist University Press, 1999).

8. Official Transcript of the American Military Tribunal in the Matter of the United States of America, against Karl Brandt, et al., Defendants, Sitting at Nurnberg, Germany, on 5 December 1946, 1015–1200 hours, Justice Beal Presiding, Harvard Law School Nuremberg Trials Project, December 5, 1946, http://nuremberg .law.harvard.edu/transcripts/1-transcript-for-nmt-1-medical-case?seq=1&q= +type:transcripts.

9. Telford Taylor, Opening Statement in the Doctors Trial by Brigadier General Telford Taylor, *Famous World Trails: Nuremberg Trials, 1945–1949*, University of Missouri, Kansas City, December 9, 1946, http://law2.umkc.edu/faculty/projects /ftrials/nuremberg/doctoropen.html.

10. Jon M. Harkness, "Nuremberg and the Issue of Wartime Experiments on US Prisoners: The Green Committee," *JAMA* 276, no. 20 (November 1996): 1672–75, https://doi.org/10.1001/jama.1996.03540200058032.

11. George J. Annas and Michael A. Grodin, eds., *The Nazi Doctors and the Nuremberg Code: Human Rights in Experimentation* (New York: Oxford University Press, 1992); Andrew C. Ivy, "The History and Ethics of the Use of Human Subjects in Medical Experiments," *Science* 108, no. 2792 (July 1948): 1–5, https://doi.org /10.1126/science.108.2792.1; Paul J. Weindling, *Nazi Medicine and the Nuremberg Trials: From Medical War Crimes to Informed Consent* (London: Palgrave Macmillian, 2004); and Evelyne Shuster, "Fifty Years Later: The Significance of the Nuremberg Code," *New England Journal of Medicine* 337, no. 20 (November 1997): 1436–40, https://doi.org/10.1056/nejm199711133372006.

12. Shuster, 1438.

13. Leo Alexander, "Ethics of Human Experimentation," *Psychiatric Journal of the University of Ottawa* 1, nos. 1–2 (January 1977): 40–46, http://psycnet.apa.org /record/1978-23763-001.

14. Mitscherlich and Mielke, *Doctors of Infamy*.

15. Leo Alexander, "Medical Science under Dictatorship," *New England Journal of Medicine* 241, no. 2 (July 1949): 39–47, https://doi.org/10.1056/NEJM194907142410201.

16. Heinrich von Staden, "'In a Pure and Holy Way': Personal and Professional Conduct in the Hippocratic Oath?," *Journal of the History of Medicine and Allied Sciences* 51, no. 4 (October 1, 1996): 406–8, https://doi.org/10.1093/jhmas/51.4.404.

17. "Nuremberg Code," US Holocaust Memorial Museum, October 1946–April 1949, https://www.ushmm.org/information/exhibitions/online-exhibitions/special -focus/doctors-trial/nuremberg-code.

18. Nuremberg Military Tribunals, Closing Argument for the United States of America, Military Tribunal No. I, C/SE No. 1, U.S. v. Karl Brandt, et al., Harvard Law School Nuremberg Trials Project, July 14, 1947, http://nuremberg.law.harvard.edu/documents/2-argument-prosecution-closing-argument?q=%2A#p.1.

19. Tatsuo Kuroyanagi, "Historical Transition in Medical Ethics—Challenges of the World Medical Association," *Japan Medical Association Journal* 56, no. 4 (July–August 2013): 220–26, http://www.med.or.jp/english/journal/pdf/2013_04/220_226.pdf.

20. *World Medical Association Bulletin* 1, no. 1 (1949): 3–14.

21. WMA, *Declaration of Geneva*, September 1948, https://www.wma.net/policies-post/wma-declaration-of-geneva/.

22. Article IV: Convention Respecting the Laws and Customs of War on Land, in "Laws of War: Laws and Customs of War on Land (Hague IV) [The Hague Convention]," *The Avalon Project: Documents in Law, History and Diplomacy,* Yale Law School, October 18, 1907, http://avalon.law.yale.edu/20th_century/hague04.asp (my emphasis).

23. Andreas Frewer, "Human Rights from the Nuremberg Doctors Trial to the Geneva Declaration: Persons and Institutions in Medical Ethics and History," *Medicine Health Care and Philosophy* 13, no. 3 (August 2010): 259–68, https://doi.org/10.1007/s11019-010-9247-2.

24. WMA, *International Code of Medical Ethics*, October 1949, https://www.wma.net/policies-post/wma-international-code-of-medical-ethics/international-code-of-medical-ethics-2006/.

25. William E. Seidelman, "Whither Nuremberg? Medicine's Continuing Nazi Heritage," *Medicine and Global Survival* 2, no. 3 (October 1995): 148–56, https://www.ippnw.org/pdf/mgs/2-3-seidelman.pdf.

26. Winfield W. Reifler, "Our Economic Contribution to Victory," *Foreign Affairs* 26, no. 1 (October 1947): 90–103, https://doi.org/10.2307/20030091.

27. Annie Jacobsen, *Operation Paperclip: The Secret Intelligence Program That Brought Nazi Scientists to America* (New York: Little, Brown, 2014).

28. Fiona McClenaghan, "British Responses to Nazi Medical War Crimes," in *Human Medical Research*, ed. Jan Schildmann, Verena Sandow, Oliver Rauprich, and Jochen Vollmann (Basel, Switzerland: Springer Basel, 2012), 7–17.

29. Lucette Lagnado, "A Scientist's Nazi-Era Past Haunts Prestigious Space Prize," *Wall Street Journal*, December 1, 2012; and "Hubertus Strughold—'Father of Space Medicine,' But at What Cost?," dirdeklein.net, November 5, 2016, https://dirkdeklein.net/2016/11/05/hubertus-strughold-father-of-space-medicinebut-at-what-cost/.

30. Paul J. Amoroso and Lynn L. Wenge, "The Human Volunteer in Military Biomedical Research," in *Military Medical Ethics*, ed. Thomas E. Beam and Linette R. Sparacino (Washington, DC: Government Printing Office, 2003), 2:436.

31. Jonathan Moreno, *Undue Risk: Secret State Experiments on Humans* (New York: Routledge, 2013): 56–57.

32. Rael D. Strous and Morris C. Edelman, "Eponyms and the Nazi Era: Time to Remember and Time for Change," *Israel Medical Association Journal* 9, no. 3 (2007): 207–14.

33. Sheldon H. Harris, *Factories of Death: Japanese Biological Warfare, 1932–1945, and the American Cover Up*, 2nd ed. (New York: Routledge, 2002); Peter Williams and David Wallace, *Unit 731: Japan's Secret Biological Warfare in World War II* (New York: Free Press, 1989); and Takashi Tsuchiya, "Ethical Lessons from Unit 731's Human Experiments" (8th World Congress of Bioethics, Beijing, China, August 8, 2006), http://www.lit.osaka-cu.ac.jp/user/tsuchiya/gyoseki/presentation/IAB8.pdf.

34. Jacobsen, *Operation Paperclip*, 348–63.

35. Dan Plesch, *Human Rights after Hitler: The Lost History of Prosecuting Axis War Crimes* (Washington, DC: Georgetown University Press, 2017).

36. Norbert Frei, *Adenauer's Germany and the Nazi Past: The Politics of Amnesty and Integration* (New York: Columbia University Press, 2002).

37. "United Nations War Crimes Commission—Central Registry of War Criminals and Security Suspects (CROWCASS), Allied Control Authority Wanted Lists Nos.: 12–13, A-Z / (Restricted)–17246," UN Archives, September 30, 1946, https://search.archives.un.org/unwcc-central-registry-of-war-criminals-and-security-suspects-crowcass-allied-control-authority-wanted-lists-nos-12–13-z-restricted.

38. "Nuremberg Trial Proceedings Volume 2: Second Day: Wednesday, 21 November 1945," *The Avalon Project: Documents in Law, History, and Diplomacy*, Yale Law School, November 21, 1945, http://avalon.law.yale.edu/imt/11-21-45.asp.

## Chapter 6. A Global Map of Torture Doctors

1. BMA, *The Torture Report: Report of a Working Party of the British Medical Association Investigating the Involvement of Doctors in Torture* (London: BMA, 1986), 1–34.

2. Freedom House, *World's Most Repressive Societies*, 2012, https://freedomhouse.org/report/special-reports/worst-worst-2012-worlds-most-repressive-societies; and Committee to Protect Journalists, *Ten Most Censored Countries*, 2015, https://cpj.org/2015/04/10-most-censored-countries.php.

3. Albanian Human Rights Group, Center for Legal Civic Initiatives, and Children's Human Rights Centre of Albania, *State Violence in Albania: An Alternative Report to the UN Committee Against Torture* (Geneva: World Organization Against Torture, 2005), 116, http://www.univie.ac.at/bimtor/dateien/albania_omct_2005_state_violence_in_albania.pdf.

4. Azerbaijan Human Rights Centre, International League for Human Rights, and the World Organization Against Torture, *Compliance of the Republic of Azerbaijan with the Convention Against Torture and Other Cruel, Inhuman or Degrading Treatment and Punishment*, May 16, 2003, 12, 22, http://www.refworld.org/docid/46c190230.html.

5. Committee Solidarity, Legal Initiative, Belarusian Helsinki Committee, and Legal Transformation Centre, *Republic of Belarus: NGO Report on the Implementation of the Convention against Torture and Other Cruel, Inhuman or Degrading Treatment or Punishment by the Republic of Belarus, in Relation to the Review of Belarus at the 47th Session of the United Nations Committee Against Torture*, 2011, 20, http://www2.ohchr.org/english/bodies/cat/docs/ngos/NGOCoalition_Belarus47_en.pdf.

6. Council of Europe Committee for the Prevention of Torture (CPT), *Report to the Bulgarian Government on the Visit to Bulgaria Carried Out by the European Committee for the Prevention of Torture and Inhuman or Degrading Treatment or Punishment (CPT) from 17 to 26 April 2002*, CPT/Inf (2004) 21, June 24, 2004, https://rm.coe.int/CoERMPublicCommonSearchServices/DisplayDCTMContent?documentId=0900001680694040.

7. CPT, *Report to the United Nations Interim Administration in Kosovo (UNMIK) on the Visit to Kosovo Carried Out by the European Committee for the Prevention of Torture and Inhuman or Degrading Treatment or Punishment (CPT) from 21 to 29 March 2007*, CPT/Inf (2009) 3, January 20, 2009, https://rm.coe.int/168069727c.

8. Vincent Iacopino, *Ending Impunity: The Use of Forensic Medical Evaluations to Document Torture and Ill Treatment in Kyrgyzstan* (New York: PHR, 2012), http://physiciansforhumanrights.org/library/reports/ending-impunity-forensic-medical-evaluations-in-kyrgyzstan.html.

9. CPT, *Report to the Government of 'the Former Yugoslav Republic of Macedonia' on the Visit to 'the Former Yugoslav Republic of Macedonia' Carried Out by the European Committee for the Prevention of Torture and Inhuman or Degrading Treatment or Punishment (CPT) from 21 to 24 November 2011*, CPT/Inf (2012) 38, December 20, 2012, 22–34, https://rm.coe.int/09000016806974dd.

10. UN General Assembly, Report of the Special Rapporteur on Torture and Other Cruel, Inhuman or Degrading Treatment or Punishment, Juan E. Méndez, A/HRC/19/61/Add.3 (March 1, 2012), 362, https://www.ohchr.org/documents/hrbodies/hrcouncil/regularsession/session19/a.hrc.19.61.add.3_efsonly.pdf.

11. Jerzy Umiastowski, "Torture in Poland," *Journal of Medical Ethics* 17 (1991): S41, https://doi.org/10.1136/jme.17.suppl.41.

12. UN General Assembly, Report of the Special Rapporteur on Torture, 117; and UN Economic and Social Council, Report of the Special Rapporteur on the Question of Torture, Sir Nigel S. Rodley, Submitted Pursuant to Commission on Human Rights resolution 1999/32, E/CN.4/2000/9/Add.3 (November 23, 1999), http://www.refworld.org/pdfid/3ae6b0970.pdf.

13. CPT, *Report to the Ukrainian Government on the Visit to Ukraine Carried Out by the European Committee for the Prevention of Torture and Inhuman or Degrading Treatment or Punishment (CPT) from 29 November to 6 December 2011*, CPT/Inf (2012) 30, November 14, 2012, https://rm.coe.int/1680698448.

14. UN Economic and Social Council, Report of the Special Rapporteur on the Question of Torture, Theo van Boven, Submitted in Accordance with Commission Resolution 2002/38, E/CN.4/2003/68/Add.2 (February 3, 2003), http://www.refworld.org/publisher,UNCHR,MISSION,,4090ffc80,0.html.

15. Coalition Against Torture and Impunity, *NGO Report on Tajikistan's Implementation of the Convention against Torture and Other Cruel, Inhuman or Degrading Treatment or Punishment*, October 12, 2012, http://www2.ohchr.org/english/bodies/cat/docs/ngos/CATI_Tajikistan_CAT49.pdf.

16. UN Economic and Social Council, Question of the Human Rights of All Persons Subjected to Any Form of Detention or Imprisonment, in Particular: Torture and Other Cruel, Inhuman or Degrading Treatment or Punishment: Report of the

Special Rapporteur, Mr. Nigel S. Rodley, Submitted Pursuant to Commission on Human Rights Resolution 1992/32, E/CN.4/1995/34 (January 12, 1995), 115, http://www.refworld.org/docid/4d3943f72.html.

17. UN General Assembly, Report of the Special Rapporteur on Torture and Other Cruel, Inhuman or Degrading Treatment or Punishment, Manfred Nowak: Mission to Kazakhstan, A/HRC/13/39/Add.3 (December 16, 2009), 48–49, https://www2.ohchr.org/english/bodies/hrcouncil/docs/13specialsession/A.HRC.13.39.Add.3_en.pdf.

18. Albanian Rehabilitation Centre for Trauma and Torture (ARCT), *Alternative Report to the List of Issues to Be Taken Up in Connection with the Consideration of the Second Periodic Report of Albania, Adopted by the Committee at Its 106th Session (October 15–November 2)*, 2013, 48, https://www.ecoi.net/en/file/local/1215958/1930_1375965413_arct-abania-hrc108.pdf.

19. CPT, *Report to the Latvian Government on the Visit to Latvia Carried Out by the European Committee for the Prevention of Torture and Inhuman or Degrading Treatment or Punishment (CPT) from 5 to 15 September 2011*, CPT/Inf (2013) 20, August 27, 2013, 31, https://rm.coe.int/1680697314.

20. Robert van Voren, "Political Abuse of Psychiatry—An Historical Overview," *Schizophrenia Bulletin* 36, no. 1 (2010): 33–35, https://doi.org/10.1093/schbul/sbp119; *Abuse of Psychiatry in the Soviet Union: Hearing Before the Subcommittee on Human Rights and International Organizations of the House Committee on Foreign Affairs and the Commission on Security and Cooperation in Europe*, 98th Cong. (1983), https://www.csce.gov/sites/helsinkicommission.house.gov/files/Abuse%20of%20Psychiatry%20in%20the%20Soviet%20Union.pdf; Carl Gershman, "Psychiatric Abuse in the Soviet Union," *Society* 21, no. 5 (July 1984): 54–59; Bloch and Reddaway, *Russia's Political Hospitals*; Anatoly Koryagin, "Unwilling Patients," *Lancet* 317, no. 8224 (1981): 821–24, https://doi.org/10.1016/S0140-6736(81)92691-X; Stover and Nightingale, *Breaking of Bodies and Minds*, 129–223; Charles J. Brown and Armando M. Lago, *The Politics of Psychiatry in Revolutionary Cuba* (New Brunswick, NJ: Transaction, 1991); Rejali, *Torture and Democracy*, 392–715; Amnesty International, *Prisoners of Conscience in Yugoslavia*, EUR 48/020/1985, January 1, 1985, https://www.amnesty.org/en/documents/EUR48/020/1985/en/; and Anatoly Koryagin, "The Involvement of Soviet Psychiatry in the Persecution of Dissenters," *British Journal of Psychiatry* 154, no. 3 (March 1989): 336–40, https://doi.org/10.1192/bjp.154.3.336.

21. Database Center for North Korean Human Rights and North Korean Human Rights Archives, *Political Prison Camps in North Korea Today*, 2011, http://rageuniversity.com/prisonescape/uk%20anti-terror%20law/Poltical-Prison-Camps-in-North-Korea.pdf.

22. Simon Tisdall, "Witness Reveals Horror of North Korean Gulag," *Guardian*, July 18, 2002, https://www.theguardian.com/world/2002/jul/19/northkorea.

23. CPT, *Report to the Croatian Government on the Visit to Croatia Carried Out by the European Committee for the Prevention of Torture and Inhuman or Degrading Treatment or Punishment (CPT) from 19 to 27 September 2012*, CPT/Inf (2014) 9, March 18, 2014, https://rm.coe.int/0900001680695591.

24. CPT, *Report to the UN Interim Administration in Kosovo*, para. 44.
25. Benito Morentin, Luis F. Callado, and M. Itaxso Idoyaga, "A Follow-up Study of Allegations of Ill-Treatment/Torture in Incommunicado Detainees in Spain: Failure of International Preventive Mechanisms," *Torture* 18, no. 2 (February 2008): 87–98, https://irct.org/assets/uploads/1018–8185_2008–2_87–98.pdf.
26. CPT, *Report to the Spanish Government on the Visit to Spain Carried Out by the European Committee for the Prevention of Torture and Inhuman or Degrading Treatment or Punishment (CPT) from 19 to 22 June 2012*, CPT/Inf (2013) 8, April 30, 2012, https://rm.coe.int/1680697ec0.
27. CPT, *Report to the Spanish Government on the Visit to Spain Carried Out by the European Committee for the Prevention of Torture and Inhuman or Degrading Treatment or Punishment (CPT) from 19 September to 1 October 2007*, CPT/Inf (2011) 11, March 25, 2011, https://rm.coe.int/0900001680697ea6; CPT, *Report to the Spanish Government on the Visit to Spain Carried Out by the European Committee for the Prevention of Torture and Inhuman or Degrading Treatment or Punishment (CPT) from 10 to 14 June 1994*, CPT/Inf (96) 9 [Part 3], March 5, 1996, https://rm.coe.int/0900001680697dec; CPT, *Report to the Spanish Government on the Visit to Spain Carried Out by the European Committee for the Prevention of Torture and Inhuman or Degrading Treatment or Punishment (CPT) from 10 to 22 April 1994*, CPT/Inf (96) 9 [Part 2], March 5, 1996, https://rm.coe.int/0900001680697dea; CPT, *Report to the Spanish Government on the Visit to Spain Carried Out by the European Committee for the Prevention of Torture and Inhuman or Degrading Treatment or Punishment (CPT) from 22 November to 4 December 1998*, CPT/Inf (2000) 5, April 13, 2000, https://rm.coe.int/0900001680697e87; and CPT, *Report to the Spanish Government on the Visit to Spain Carried Out by the European Committee for the Prevention of Torture and Inhuman or Degrading Treatment or Punishment (CPT) from 31 May to 13 June 2011*, CPT/Inf (2013) 6, April 30, 2013, https://rm.coe.int/09000016806cb01c.
28. CPT, *Report to the Spanish Government on the Visit to Spain Carried Out by the European Committee for the Prevention of Torture and Inhuman or Degrading Treatment or Punishment (CPT) from 17 to 18 January 1997*, CPT/Inf (2000) 3, April 13, 2000, 9–10, https://rm.coe.int/0900001680697e69.
29. Leonard A. Sagan and Albert Jonsen, "Medical Ethics and Torture," *New England Journal of Medicine* 294, no. 26 (June 1976): 1427–30, https://doi.org/10.1056/nejm197606242942605.
30. CPT, *Report to the Portuguese Government on the Visit to Portugal Carried Out by the European Committee for the Prevention of Torture and Inhuman or Degrading Treatment or Punishment (CPT) from 14 to 26 May 1995*, CPT/Inf (1996) 31, November 21, 1996, https://rm.coe.int/0900001680697950; CPT, *Report to the Portuguese Government on the Visit to Portugal Carried Out by the European Committee for the Prevention of Torture and Inhuman or Degrading Treatment or Punishment (CPT) from 20 to 24 October 1996*, CPT/Inf (1998) 1, January 13, 1998, https://rm.coe.int/09000016806979af; CPT, *Report to the Portuguese Government on the Visit to Portugal Carried Out by the European Committee for the Prevention*

*of Torture and Inhuman or Degrading Treatment or Punishment (CPT) from 17 to 20 December 2002*, CPT/Inf (2007) 11, January 25, 2007, https://rm.coe.int /09000016806979b4; and CPT, *Report to the Portuguese Government on the Visit to Portugal Carried Out by the European Committee for the Prevention of Torture and Inhuman or Degrading Treatment or Punishment (CPT) from 13 to 17 May 2013*, CPT/Inf (2013) 35, November 26, 2013, https://rm.coe.int/09000016806979c5.

31. Rejali, *Torture and Democracy*, 47.

32. Adam Nossiter, "French Soldiers Tortured Algerians, Macron Admits Six Decades Later," *New York Times*, September 13, 2018, https://www.nytimes.com /2018/09/13/world/europe/france-algeria-maurice-audin.html.

33. Frederick Taylor, *Exorcising Hitler: The Occupation and Denazification of Germany* (London: Bloomsbury Press, 2013).

34. Alexander Dückers, "Nazi War Crimes and Medicine 50 Years On," *Lancet* 349, no. 9055 (March 1997): 886, https://doi.org/10.1016/s0140–6736(05)61802–8.

35. Horst H. Freyhofer, *The Nuremberg Medical Trial: The Holocaust and the Origin of the Nuremberg Medical Code*, 2nd ed. (New York: Peter Lang Publishing, 2005), https://free-ebooks.com/ebooks/the-nuremberg-medical-trial-the-holocaust -and-the-origin-of-the-nuremberg-medical-code-studies-in-modern-european -history-v-53-horst-h-freyhofer/.

36. Kulish and Mekhennet, *Eternal Nazi*.

37. Robert S. Wistrich, "Werner Heyde," in *Who's Who in Nazi Germany* (New York: Routledge, 2001), 107.

38. Seidelman, "Whither Nuremberg?," 148–57.

39. "Ex-Nazi Officer Admits Passing Order to Kill All Jews in Pinsk," Jewish Telegraphic Agency, February 18, 1964, https://www.jta.org/1964/02/18/archive/ex -nazi-officer-admits-passing-order-to-kill-all-jews-in-pinsk.

40. Lawrence W. White, "The Nazi Doctors and the Medical Community: Honor or Censure? The Case of Hans Sewering," *Journal of Medical Humanities* 17, no. 2 (June 1996): 119–35, https://doi.org/10.1007/BF02276813; and Michael A. Grodin, George J. Annas, and Leonard H. Glantz, "Medicine and Human Rights: A Proposal for International Action," *Hastings Center Report* 23, no. 4 (July 1993): 8–12, https://doi.org/10.2307/3562583.

41. William E. Seidelman, "From the Danube to the Spree: Deception, Truth and Morality in Medicine," in *Jahrbuch 1999* [Yearbook 1999], ed. Siegwald Ganglmair (Vienna: Documentationsarchiv des Österreichischen Widerstanders, 1999), 15–32, http://www.doew.at/erforschen/publikationen/gesamtverzeichnis/jahrbuch /jahrbuch-1999-schwerpunkt-euthanasie-ns-medizin.

42. Harry de Quetteville, "German Doctor 'Who Sent 900 Children to Nazi Camp' Honoured," *Telegraph*, May 25, 2008, https://www.telegraph.co.uk/news /worldnews/2027938/German-doctor-who-sent-900-children-to-Nazi-camp -honoured.html; and Allan Hall, "Germans Give Former SS Doctor Accused of Killing 900 Children a Medal," *Daily Mail*, May 25, 2008, http://www.dailymail .co.uk/news/article-1021807/Germans-SS-doctor-accused-killing-900-children -medal.html.

43. Annette Tuffs, "Obituary of Past President of German Medical Association Omits Details of Nazi Past, Medical Historians Say," *British Medical Journal* 341 (August 2010): 4468, https://doi.org/10.1136/bmj.c4468.

44. German Medical Association, "Nuremberg Declaration of the German Medical Assembly 2012," in Steven Kolb, Paul Weindling, Volker Roelcke, and Horst Seithe, "Apologising for Nazi Medicine: A Constructive Starting Point," *Lancet* 380, no. 9483 (August 25, 2012): 722–23, https://doi.org/10.1016/S0140–6736(12)61396–8.

45. Tobias Voigt and Peter Erler, *Medizin hinter Gittern: Das Stasi-Haftkrankenhaus in Berlin-Hohenschönhausen* [Medicine behind bars: The Stasi prison hospital in Berlin-Hohenschönhausen] (Berlin: Jaron Verlag, 2011); and Solveig Grothe, "Stasi-Haftlinik-Der Feind auf dem OP-Tisch" [Stasi prison hospital: The enemy on the operating table], *Spiegel Online*, November 29, 2011, http://www.spiegel.de/einestages/stasi-haftklinik-a-947401.html.

46. Human Rights Watch, *The Torture of Tasneem Khalil: How the Bangladesh Military Abuses Its Power under the State of Emergency*, February 13, 2008, https://www.hrw.org/report/2008/02/13/torture-tasneem-khalil/how-bangladesh-military-abuses-its-power-under-state; and Ian Cobain and Fariha Karim, "Bangladeshi MP 'Tortured' by British-Trained Paramilitary Unit," *Guardian*, February 25, 2011, https://www.theguardian.com/law/2011/feb/25/bangladeshi-mp-tortured-rapid-action-battalion.

47. Tarique Anwar, "Gross Violation of Human Rights in Bhopal Jail: SIMI Under Trials Suffer Violence, Torture and Religious Discrimination," *News Click*, April 2, 2018, https://newsclick.in/gross-violation-human-rights-bhopal-jail-simi-undertrials-suffer-violence-torture-and-religious; "India: Threatened with Violence for Reporting Torture to Police," Asian Human Rights Commission, August 7, 2012, http://www.humanrights.asia/news/urgent-appeals/AHRC-UAU-026–2012; and Varinder Bhatia, "Second Autopsy Finds 14 Injuries Caused by 'Brutal Assault,'" *Indian Express*, November 28, 2013, http://archive.indianexpress.com/news/second-autopsy-finds-14-injuries-caused-by—brutal-assault-/1200545/.

48. Reis et al., "Physician Participation," 1480–86; and Human Rights Watch, *"No One Is Safe": Abuses of Women in Iraq's Criminal Justice System*, February 2014, 19–37, https://www.hrw.org/sites/default/files/reports/iraq0214webwcover.pdf.

49. Human Rights Watch, *Jordan: Torture and Impunity in Jordan's Prisons: Reforms Fail to Tackle Widespread Abuse*, October 8, 2008, https://www.hrw.org/report/2008/10/08/torture-and-impunity-jordans-prisons/reforms-fail-tackle-widespread-abuse; and Amnesty International, *Jordan: "Your Confessions Are Ready for You to Sign": Detention and Torture of Political Suspects*, MDE 16/005/2006, July 23, 2006, https://www.amnesty.org/en/documents/mde16/005/2006/en/.

50. "Burma: Police Torture Man to Death, Detain Mother, and Obstruct Justice," Asian Human Rights Commission, October 2, 2012, http://www.humanrights.asia/news/urgent-appeals/AHRC-UAC-176–2012; Assistance Association for Political Prisoners (Burma), *The Darkness We See: Torture in Burma's Interrogation Centers and Prisons*, December 2005, 9, 85, http://aappb.org/wp/tortour_report.pdf;

"Burma/Myanmar: The Police Cannot Avoid Responsibility for the Torture to Death of a Man in Custody," Asian Human Rights Commission, March 17, 2014, http://www.humanrights.asia/news/urgent-appeals/AHRC-UAU-010–2014.

51. "Nepal: Torture of an 18-Year-Old Student by the Police in Jhapa District," Asian Human Rights Commission, August 1, 2012, http://www.humanrights.asia/news /urgent-appeals/AHRC-UAC-137–2012; UN General Assembly, Report of the Special Rapporteur, A/HRC/19/61/Add.3.

52. UN General Assembly, Report of the Special Rapporteur, A/HRC/19/61/Add.3.

53. "Philippines: Torture Victims Speak Out—'The Evidence Is Suppressed to Weaken a Case,'" Asian Human Rights Commission, June 17, 2011, http://www .humanrights.asia/opinions/interviews/AHRC-ETC-028–2011; "Philippines: Torture Victims Whose Complaints of Injuries Were Ignored by Doctors Had Their Case Dismissed," Asian Human Rights Commission, January 31, 2012, http://www.humanrights.asia/news/urgent-appeals/AHRC-UAU-003–2012/; "Philippines: Investigate Two Separate Incidents of Torture in Basilan," Asian Human Rights Commission, September 23, 2011, http://www.humanrights .asia/news/urgent-appeals/AHRC-UAC-174–2011; and June Pagaduan-Lopez, "Medical Professionals and Human Rights in the Philippines," *Journal of Medical Ethics* 17 (December 1991): S42–50, https://doi.org/10.1136/jme.17.suppl.42.

54. UN General Assembly, Report of the Special Rapporteur, A/HRC/19/61/Add.3; "Medical Colluding with Police Refuse to Treat a Victim Tortured by Ingiriya Police," Sri Lanka Brief, November 6, 2017, http://srilankabrief.org/2017/06 /sri-lanka-medical-officers-colluding-with-police-refuse-to-treat-a-victim-tortured -by-ingiriya-police/; "Sri Lanka: Officers of the Karandeniya Police Torture and Threaten to Sodomize Businessman, Insulting Him about His 'Low' Caste Origin," Asian Human Rights Commission, June 10, 2013, http://www.humanrights .asia/news/ahrc-news/AHRC-STM-106–2013; "Sri Lanka: Young Man Beaten Brutally and Laid with Fabricated Charges," Asian Human Rights Commission, January 24, 2011, http://www.humanrights.asia/news/urgent-appeals/AHRC-UAC -045–2011; "Sri Lanka: Failure of Medical Examination in a Case of Police Torture," Asian Human Rights Commission, May 5, 2009, http://www.humanrights .asia/news/urgent-appeals/AHRC-UAC-046–2009; "Sri Lanka: Police, Doctors and Magistrates Are Complicit in a Man's Torture," Asian Human Rights Commission, December 1, 2009, http://www.humanrights.asia/news/urgent-appeals/AHRC -UAC-166–2009; and Lewis Davis, "Sri Lanka's Judicial Medical Officers, Their Concerns and the Torture Shortcut," Asian Human Rights Commission, April 2010, http://www.humanrights.asia/resources/journals-magazines/eia/eiav4n2/sri -lankas-judicial-medical-officers-their-concerns-and-the-torture-shortcut.

55. Desmond de Silva et al., *A Report into the Credibility of Certain Evidence with Regard to Torture and Execution of Persons Incarcerated by the Current Syrian Regime* (London: Carter-Ruck, January 2014), https://static.guim.co.uk/ni/1390226674736 /syria-report-execution-tort.pdf; "Sri Lanka: Failure of Medical Examination."

56. Amnesty International, *Thailand: Submission to the United Nations Committee Against Torture*, ASA 39/003/2014, April 11, 2014, https://www.amnesty.org /en/documents/ASA39/003/2014/en/; Cross Cultural Foundation, Duayjai,

and Patani Human Rights Organization, *Torture and Ill Treatment in Thailand's Deep South*, August 26, 2016, http://alrc.asia/article2/2016/08/torture-and-Ill -Treatment-in-thailands-deep-south/.

57. Human Rights Watch, *Public Insecurity: Deaths in Custody and Police Brutality in Vietnam*, September 16, 2014, https://www.hrw.org/report/2014/09/16/public -insecurity/deaths-custody-and-police-brutality-vietnam.

58. Alkarama, *Kuwait: Alternative Report Submitted to the Committee Against Torture in the Context of the Review of the Second Periodic Report of Kuwait*, 2011, http:// tbinternet.ohchr.org/Treaties/CAT/Shared%20Documents/KWT/INT_CAT _NGO_KWT_46_9455_E.pdf; and Alarkama, *Kuwait: Torture and Ill-Treatment of Mr. Al-Dhafeery*, 2008, http://en.alkarama.org/kuwait/119-kuwait-torture-and -Ill-Treatment-of-mr-al-dhafeery.

59. Jagdish C. Sobti, B. C. Chapparaawal, and Erik Holst, "Study of Knowledge, Attitude, and Practices concerning Aspects of Torture," *Journal of the Indian Medical Association* 98, no. 6 (2000): 334–35, 338–39.

60. Ugur Cilasun, "Torture and the Participation of Doctors," *Journal of Medical Ethics* 17 (December 1991): S21–22, https://www.ncbi.nlm.nih.gov/pmc/articles /PMC1378166/; Yasmin Naqvi, *Rights of the Child in Turkey*, ed. Roberta Cecchetti (Geneva: World Organization Against Torture, 2001), http://www.omct.org /files/2001/06/2103/turkeycc06.01.pdf; International Rehabilitation Council for Torture Victims, "In Prison for Protecting Torture Victims in Turkey," May 2010, https://irct.org/media-and-resources/latest-news/article/572; Yasemin N. Oguz and Steven H. Miles, "The Physician and Prison Hunger Strikes: Reflecting on the Experience in Turkey," *Journal of Medical Ethics* 31, no. 3 (2005): 169–72, https:// doi.org/10.1136/jme.2004.006973; and Somini Sengupta, "A Turkish Doctor's Specialty: The Torture Victim," *New York Times*, January 26, 2002, https://www .nytimes.com/2002/01/26/world/the-saturday-profile-a-turkish-doctor-s-specialty -the-torture-victim.htm.

61. Pagaduan-Lopez, "Medical Professionals," 42–50.

62. Hadas Ziv, *Physicians and Torture: The Case of Israel* (Tel Aviv: PHR–Israel, September 2000), https://www.scribd.com/document/42632666/Physicians-for-Human -Rights-Israel-Physicians-and-Torture-The-Case-of-Israel-September-2000; Amnesty International, *Israel and the Occupied Territories: "Under Constant Medical Supervision": Torture, Ill-Treatment and the Health Professionals in Israel and the Occupied Territories*, MDE 15/037/1996, August 13, 1996, https://www.amnesty .org/en/documents/MDE15/037/1996/en/; International Rehabilitation Council for Torture Victims (IRCT), "Forensic Evidence in the Fight against Torture: Concurrent Panels," *Human Rights Brief* 19, no. 4 (2012): 30–31; Yudkin, "Israeli Medical Association," 4078; Noga Kadman, *Backed by the System: Abuse and Torture at the Shikma Interrogation Facility* (Jerusalem: B'Tselem, HaMoked Center for the Defense of the Individual, and the European Union, 2015), https://www .btselem.org/sites/default/files2/201512_backed_by_the_system_eng.pdf; Public Committee Against Torture in Israel (PCATI) and PHR–Israel, *Doctoring the Evidence, Abandoning the Victim: The Involvement of Medical Professionals in Torture and Ill Treatment in Israel*, October 2011, http://stoptorture.org.il/wp-content/uploads

/2015/10/Doctoring-the-Evidence-Abandoning-the-Victim_November2011.pdf; PCATI, Adalah–The Legal Center for Arab Minority Rights in Israel, Al Mezan Center for Human Rights, and PHR–Israel, *NGO Report to the UN Human Rights Committee Prior to the Adoption of List of Issues for Israel,* June 4, 2012, https://www.adalah.org/uploads/oldfiles/Public/files/English/International_Advocacy/Torture_HRC%20LOIPR%203%206%202012.pdf; WMA, IMA, Dr. Yoram Blachar, and Torture in Israel, "Factsheet 54," Canadians for Justice and Peace in the Middle East, February 2009, http://www.cjpme.org/fs_054; and Derek Summerfield, "Medical Ethics, the Israeli Medical Association, and the State of the World Medical Association: Open Letter to the BMA," *British Medical Journal* 327, no. 7414 (September 2003): 561, http://www.bmj.com/content/327/7414/561.1.

63. Yudkin, "Israeli Medical Association," 4078.

64. Amnesty International, *Algeria: Unrestrained Powers: Torture by Algeria's Military Security,* MDE 28/004/2006, July 9, 2006, 34–36, https://www.amnesty.org/en/search/?q=MDE+28%2F004%2F2006.

65. "Ahmed Cherbi, Abducted and Tortured in 2002 to Confirm the Official Version of the Assassination of Lounès Matoub," Algeria-Watch, December 13, 2009, https://algeria-watch.org/?p=4174.

66. "The Case of the 'Islamists': Torture in the Name of the Fight against Terrorism," International Federation for Human Rights (FIDH), March 28, 2008, https://www.fidh.org/en/region/Africa/mauritania/The-Case-of-the-Islamists-Torture.

67. Alkarama, *Morocco: Follow-up to the Recommendations of the Committee Against Torture in the Context of the Fourth Periodic Review of Morocco,* October 1, 2012, http://tbinternet.ohchr.org/Treaties/CAT/Shared%20Documents/MAR/INT_CAT_NGS_MAR_12396_E.pdf.

68. Werner Menges, "Orina Made 'Torture' Claim to Doctor," *Namibian,* October 19, 2010, https://www.namibian.com.na/index.php?id=71925.

69. UN Economic and Social Council, Question of the Human Rights, E/CN.4/1995/34, 115.

70. Swaziland Democracy Campaign, South African Chapter, "It's Official: Comrade Sipho Jele Did Not Commit Suicide: He Was Murdered by Swaziland Police: Lies and Slander Fail to Persuade," press release, July 11, 2010, http://www.cosatu.org.za/docs/pr/2010/pr0711.html; and Richard Rooney, "Evidence of Swazi Police Torture," *Swazi Media Commentary* (blog), September 13, 2009, https://swazimedia.blogspot.com/2009/09/evidence-of-swazi-police-torture.html.

71. UN General Assembly, Report of the Committee Against Torture, A/55/44 (2000), http://undocs.org/en/A/55/44; Human Rights Watch, *The Administration of Justice in Tunisia: Torture, Trumped-Up Charges and a Tainted Trial,* March 2000, https://www.hrw.org/reports/2000/tunisia/; UN Committee Against Torture, Decisions of the Committee Against Torture under Article 22 of the Convention against Torture and Other Cruel, Inhuman or Degrading Treatment or Punishment: Communication No. 188/2001: Tunisia, CAT/C/31/D/188/2001 (2003), http://digitallibrary.un.org/record/506924.

72. "Yemen: Detained, Tortured, and Disappeared," Human Rights Watch, May 7, 2012, https://www.hrw.org/news/2012/05/07/yemen-detained-tortured-and

-disappeared; Dariusch Atighetchi, *Islamic Bioethics: Problems and Perspectives* (Netherlands: Springer, 2007), 60, https://link.springer.com/content/pdf/bfm %3A978-1-4020-4962-0%2F1.pdf.

73. "Zambia: Police Brutality, Torture Rife," Human Rights Watch, September 7, 2010, https://www.hrw.org/news/2010/09/07/zambia-police-brutality-torture-rife.

74. Amnesty International, *Kenya: Detention, Torture, and Health Professionals*, AFR 32/001/1997, January 8, 1997, 6, http://www.amnesty.org/en/library/info/AFR32 /001/1997/en.

75. Patrick Kingsley and Louisa Loveluck, "Egyptian Doctors Ordered to Operate on Protesters without Anaesthetic," *Guardian*, April 11, 2013, https://www.theguardian .com/world/2013/apr/11/egypt-doctors-operate-protesters-anaesthetic; John Ehab, "Journalists Protest State Media Coverage of Alexandria Police Killing," *Egypt Independent*, June 30, 2010, http://www.egyptindependent.com/journalists-protest-state -media-coverage-alexandria-police-killing; Fady Salah, "Tahrir Doctors File Complaint against FJP Member," *Daily News*, December 12, 2012, www.dailynewsegypt .com/2012/12/12/tahrir-doctors-file-complaint-against-fjp-member/; and El Shafi M. Beshir, "How to Struggle against Torture," *Journal of Medical Ethics* 17 (December 1991): S62–63, https://doi.org/10.1136/jme.17.Suppl.62.

76. Amnesty International, *Involvement of Medical Personnel in Abuses against Detainees and Prisoners*, ACT 75/008/1990, November 7, 1990, https://www.amnesty.org /en/documents/act75/008/1990/en/; and Wendy Orr, "Health Professionals in the South African Military," in *An Ambulance of the Wrong Colour: Health Professionals, Human Rights and Ethics in South Africa*, ed. Laurel Baldwin-Ragaven, Leslie London, and Jeanelle De Gruchy (Cape Town: University of Cape Town Press, 1999), 119–31.

77. Mary Rayner, *Turning a Blind Eye? Medical Accountability and the Prevention of Torture in South Africa* (Washington, DC: Committee on Scientific Freedom and Responsibility, American Association for the Advancement of Science, 2008).

78. Mikki van Zyl et al., *The Aversion Project: Human Rights Abuses of Gays and Lesbians in the South African Defence Force by Health Workers during the Apartheid Era* (Cape Town: Simply Said and Done, 1999), https://www.scribd.com/document /235770931/Aversion.

79. Leslie London et al., "Medical Complicity in Torture—Healing the Past," *South African Medical Journal* 86, no. 9 (September 1996): 1069–70, https://repository .library.georgetown.edu/handle/10822/895959; "Call for a Doctors' Truth Commission," *Mail and Guardian*, August 2, 1996, https://mg.co.za/article/1996-08 -02-call-for-a-doctors-truth-commission; Barend B. Mandell, Gavin P. Damster, and H. A. Hanekom, "MASA [Medical Association of South Africa] and a Truth Commission for the Medical Profession: Editorial Commentary and Debate," *South African Medical Journal* 86, no. 9 (1996): 1070–71, https://repository.library .georgetown.edu/handle/10822/896269.

80. Inter-American Commission on Human Rights, *Case 2759: Bolivia*, March 7, 1979, https://www.cidh.oas.org/annualrep/78eng/Bolivia.2759.htm; and Blas Valencia Campos et al., *Report No. 84/08, Petition 40–03: Admissibility: Bolivia*

(Washington, DC: Inter-American Commission on Human Rights, October 30, 2008), http://cidh.org/annualrep/2008eng/Bolivia40.03eng.htm.

81. Human Rights Watch, *Peru: Torture and Political Persecution in Peru*, December 1997, https://www.hrw.org/reports/1997/peru/.

82. Amnesty International, *Amnesty International Annual Report 1997*, POL 10/0001/1997, June 17, 1997, 332–34, https://www.amnesty.org/en/documents /pol10/0001/1997/en/; and Maolis Castro, "Torture Victims in Venezuela Testify to Maduro Regime's Brutality," trans. Nick Lyne, *El País*, August 10, 2017, https://elpais.com/elpais/2017/08/10/inenglish/1502361209_348789.html.

83. Adam Nossiter, "Islamists' Harsh Justice Is on the Rise in North Mali," *New York Times*, December 27, 2012, https://www.nytimes.com/2012/12/28/world /africa/islamists-harsh-justice-on-rise-in-northern-mali.html; Peter Moszynski, "Sudanese Doctors' Role in Judicial Amputation 'Breaks Medical Ethics,'" *British Medical Journal* 346 (February 2013): 1253, https://doi.org/10.1136/bmj .f1253; Human Rights Watch, *"Political Shari'a": Human Rights and Islamic Law in Northern Nigeria*, September 21, 2004, https://www.hrw.org/report/2004/09/21 /political-sharia/human-rights-and-islamic-law-northern-nigeria.

84. Pierre Perrin, "Sharia Punishment, Treatment, and Speaking Out, Supporting Sharia or Providing Treatment: The International Committee of the Red Cross, Learning to Express Dissent: Médecins Sans Frontières," British Medical Journal 319, no. 7207 (August 1999): 445, https://doi.org/10.1136/bmj.319.7207.445.

85. Atighetchi, *Islamic Bioethics*, 60.

86. "Sudan: Doctors Perform Amputations for Courts," African Center for Justice and Peace Studies, February 27, 2013, http://www.acjps.org/sudan-doctors -perform-amputations-for-courts/.

87. Perrin, "Sharia Punishment," 445.

88. Adebayo Adejumo and Prisca O. Adejumo, "Time to Act against Medical Collusion in Punitive Amputations," *British Medical Journal* 330, no. 7502 (May 2005): 1277, https://doi.org/10.1136/bmj.330.7502.1277.

89. BMA, *Medicine Betrayed*, 94.

90. Human Rights Watch, "Political Shari'a"; Sam Olukoya, "Eyewitness: Nigeria's Sharia Amputees," BBC News World, December 19, 2002, http://news.bbc.co.uk /2/hi/africa/2587039.stm; and Amnesty International, *"Welcome to Hell Fire": Torture and Other Ill-Treatment in Nigeria*, AFR 44/011/2014, September 18, 2014, https://www.amnesty.org/en/documents/afr44/011/2014/en/.

91. "The Islamic Code of Medical Ethics," *World Medical Journal* 29, no. 5 (September–October 1982): 78–80.

92. Shahid Athar, "The Use of Physicians for Human Torture," Islamic Medical Association of North America, July 6, 2005, http://www.consciencelaws.org/religion /religion032.aspx.

93. Amnesty International, "Sudan: Judges to Be Trained to Carry Out Amputations," news release, March 12, 2013; and PHR, "Sudan: Doctors Perform Amputations for Courts," news release, February 27, 2013, http://physiciansforhumanrights .org/press/press-releases/sudan-doctors-perform-amputations-for-courts.html.

94. Amnesty International, "Sudan: Judges."

95. Amnesty International, *Amnesty International Report 2016/17: The State of the World's Human Rights*, 2017, 52, 193, https://www.amnesty.org/en/documents /pol10/4800/2017/en/.

96. Paulo Muoka Nzili vs. The Foreign and Commonwealth Office, HQ09X02666 (Justice Queen's Bench Division 2010), http://www.leighday.co.uk/LeighDay /media/LeighDay/documents/Mau%20Mau/Claimant%20statements/Paulo-Nzili -WS—26-10-10—-Final-.pdf.

97. Paulo Muoka Nzili v. Foreign and Commonwealth Office, Q.B. (2010); "UK to Compensate Kenya's Mau Mau Torture Victims," *Guardian*, June 6, 2013, https:// www.theguardian.com/world/2013/jun/06/uk-compensate-kenya-mau-mau -torture.

98. Lisa Durnian, "Whipping as a Criminal Punishment: Research Brief 21," Prosecution Project, March 14, 2016, https://prosecutionproject.griffith.edu.au /whipping-as-a-criminal-punishment/; South Australian Branch of the Howard League for Penal Reform, "Corporal Punishment in South Australia," *Adelaide Law Review* 6 (1963): 84–91, http://www.austlii.edu.au/au/journals/AdelLawRw /1963/6.pdf.

99. US Department of State, *Brunei: Bureau of Democracy, Human Rights, and Labor 2005*, March 8, 2006, http://www.state.gov/j/drl/rls/hrrpt/2005/61602.htm.

100. Colin Farrell, "The Canadian Prison Strap," Corpun, 2018, https://www.corpun .com/canada.htm.

101. Robert Fisk, "Scarred by the Savage Lash of Islamic Justice," *Independent*, October 13, 1995, https://www.independent.co.uk/news/world/scarred-by-the-savage -lash-of-islamic-justice-1577324.html.

102. Associated Press, "Hong Kong Is to Abolish Use of Floggings for Punishment," *New York Times*, August 24, 1989, http://www.nytimes.com/1989/08/24/world /hong-kong-is-to-abolish-use-of-floggings-for-punishment.html.

103. "Punishment of Flogging," 253 Parl. Deb. H.C. (1880) cols. 960–62, http:// hansard.millbanksystems.com/commons/1880/jun/28/india-punishment-of -flogging.

104. "Iran: Wave of Floggings, Amputations and Other Vicious Punishments," Amnesty International, January 19, 2017, https://www.amnesty.org/en/latest/news/2017/01 /iran-wave-of-floggings-amputations-and-other-vicious-punishments/.

105. Amnesty International, *Jordan: Human Rights Protection after the State of Emergency*, MDE 16/02/90 (London: Amnesty International, June 1990).

106. Colin Farrell, "Judicial Caning in Singapore, Malaysia, and Brunei," Corpun, September 2012, https://www.corpun.com/singfeat.htm#medical; and Amnesty International, *A Blow to Humanity: Torture by Judicial Caning in Malaysia*, ASA 28/013/2010, December 6, 2010, https://www.amnesty.org/en/documents/asa28 /013/2010/en/.

107. Amnesty International, *Qatar: Briefing to the United Nations Committee Against Torture*, MDE 22/001/2012, October 12, 2012, https://www.amnesty.org/en /documents/mde22/001/2012/en/; "'My Whole Back Felt like It Was on Fire': As

a British Teacher Faces 40 Lashes, One Man Speaks Out," *Daily Mail*, November 28, 2007, http://www.dailymail.co.uk/news/article-496844/My-felt-like-As -British-teacher-faces-40-lashes-man-speaks-out.html.

108. "Saudi Arabia: Doctors Find Raif Badawi Unfit for Flogging on Health Grounds Second Week in a Row," Amnesty International, January 22, 2015, https://www .amnesty.org/en/latest/news/2015/01/saudi-arabia-doctors-find-raif-badawi-unfit -flogging-health-grounds-second-week-row/.

109. Firouzeh Bahrampour, "The Caning of Michael Fay: Can Singapore's Punishment Withstand the Scrutiny of International Law?," *American University Law Review* 10, no. 3 (1995): 1075–78, http://digitalcommons.wcl.american.edu/auilr /vol10/iss3/2/.

110. Amnesty International, *Whippings: South Africa*, AFR 53/19/90 (London: Amnesty International, 1990).

111. Ibrahim Dosara, "Nigerian Teen Accepts Flogging Sentence," *Globe and Mail*, January 15, 2001, https://www.theglobeandmail.com/news/world/nigerian-teen -accepts-flogging-sentence/article1029627/.

112. Andreas Harsono, "Public Floggings in Indonesia Top 500," Human Rights Watch, October 24, 2017, https://www.hrw.org/news/2017/10/24/public-floggings -indonesia-top-500; Nurdin Hasan, "Indonesia Carries Out First-Ever Caning of Gay Couple," *Benar News* (Banda Aceh), May 23, 2017, http://www.benarnews .org/english/news/indonesian/Aceh-gay-men-caned-05232017152637.html; AFP, "Man Collapses after Caning for Breaking Sharia Law in Indonesia," *Express Tribune*, February 27, 2017, https://tribune.com.pk/story/1340744/man-collapses -caning-breaking-sharia-law-indonesia/.

113. Richard Willis, Lindsay Murdoch, and Damien Comerford, "Freedom for O'Meally," *The Age*, July 5, 1979.

114. Amnesty International, *Medical Letter-Writing Action: Whipping in Pakistan*, ASA 33/001/1990, February 23, 1990, https://www.amnesty.org/en/documents/asa33 /001/1990/en/.

115. Amnesty International, *Kenya: Detention, Torture and Health Professionals*, AFR 32/001/1997, January 8, 1997, 6–7, https://www.amnesty.org/en/documents /AFR32/001/1997/en/.

116. Amnesty International, *Blow to Humanity*, 14.

117. Amnesty International, 23.

118. BMA, *Medicine Betrayed*, 95.

119. Cody Cichowitz, Leonard Rubenstein, and Chris Beyrer, "Forced Anal Examinations to Ascertain Sexual Orientation and Sexual Behavior: An Abusive and Medically Unsound Practice," *Public Library of Science Medicine* 15, no. 3 (March 16, 2018), https://doi.org/10.1371/journal.pmed.1002536; Human Rights Watch, *Dignity Debased: Forced Anal Examinations in Homosexuality Prosecutions*, 2016, https://www.hrw.org/sites/default/files/report_pdf/globallgbtanalexams0716web .pdf; Amnesty International, *Making Love a Crime: Criminalization of Same-Sex Conduct in Sub-Saharan Africa*, AFR 01/001/2013, June 25, 2013, http://www .amnesty.org/en/library/info/AFR01/001/2013/en; UN General Assembly, Report

of the Special Rapporteur on Torture and Other Cruel, Inhuman or Degrading Treatment or Punishment, Juan E. Méndez, A/HRC/16/52/Add.1 (March 1, 2001), 59, http://www2.ohchr.org/english/bodies/hrcouncil/docs/16session/A .HRC.16.52.Add.1_EFSonly.pdf; Gianluca Mezzofiore, "Egypt: Police Arrest 14 at Health Centre for 'Practicing Homosexuality,'" *International Business Times*, October 14, 2013, http://www.ibtimes.co.uk/egypt-police-arrests-homosexuality -14-health-centre-513653; Amnesty International, "Malawi: Amnesty International Calls for the Unconditional Release of Gay Couple," news release, January, 6, 2009, https://www.amnesty.org.uk/press-releases/malawi-amnesty-calls -unconditional-release-gay-couple; Neela Ghoshal, "Teen Posted on Instagram and the Next Thing He Knew, a Doctor Was Invading His Body," *East African*, June 1, 2017, https://www.theeastafrican.co.ke/OpEd/comment/Teen-whose -Facebook-post-led-to-invasive-test/434750–3951220-item-0-bws4tmz/index .html; and "Zambian Gay Law Causes Uproar," eNews Channel Africa, September 17, 2013, http://www.enca.com/africa/amnesty-international-fights -homosexual-zambians.

120. "Submission to the United Nations Committee Against Torture on Tunisia," Human Rights Watch, April 4, 2016, https://www.hrw.org/news/2016/04 /04/submission-united-nations-committee-against-torture-tunisia; and Neela Ghoshal, "Anal Exams That 'Test' for Homosexuality Amount to Torture," *Advocate*, July 27, 2016, https://www.advocate.com/commentary/2016/7/27/anal -exams-test-homosexuality-amount-torture.

121. Nadim Houry and Graeme Reid, "It's Part of the Job: Ill-Treatment and Torture of Vulnerable Groups in Lebanese Police Stations," Human Rights Watch, June 26, 2013, https://www.hrw.org/report/2013/06/26/its-part-job/Ill-Treatment -and-torture-vulnerable-groups-lebanese-police-stations; "Outraged Lebanese Demand End to Anal Exams on Gay Men," BBC News, August 8, 2012, http:// www.bbc.com/news/world-middle-east-19166156; and Adam Withnall, "Banned Anal Exam 'Akin to Torture' Still Being Used by Police in Lebanon to Determine if People Are Gay," *Independent*, July 16, 2014, http://www.independent.co.uk/news /world/middle-east/banned-anal-exam-akin-to-torture-still-being-used-by-police -in-lebanon-to-determine-if-people-are-gay-9610309.html.

122. Afghanistan Independent Human Rights Commission (AIHRC), "Forced Gynecological Exams as Sexual Harassment and Human Rights Violation," *Open Asia*, March 4, 2016, http://openasia.org/en/?p=6610.

123. Robert Mackey, "One Year Later, Egyptian Women Subjected to 'Virginity Tests' Await Justice," *The Lede* (blog), March 9, 2012, http://thelede.blogs.nytimes.com /2012/03/09/one-year-later-egyptian-women-subjected-to-virginity-tests-await -justice/; and Ali Abdelaty, "Egypt Increases Jail Terms for People Who Perform Female Genital Mutilation," *Huffington Post*, September 29, 2016, https:// www.huffingtonpost.com/entry/egypt-approves-tougher-law-female-genital -mutilation-fgm_us_57ed2041e4b0c2407cdc1144.

124. Abdel-Rahman Hussein, "Egyptian Army Doctor Cleared over 'Virginity Tests' on Women Activists," *Guardian*, March 11, 2012, http://www.theguardian.com /world/2012/mar/11/egypt-doctor-cleared-virginity-tests.

125. WMA, *Resolution on Prohibition of Forced Anal Examinations to Substantiate Same-Sex Sexual Activity*, October 2017, https://www.wma.net/policies-post/wma -resolution-on-prohibition-of-forced-anal-examinations-to-substantiate-same -sex-sexual-activity/.

## Chapter 7. The Paradox of the United Kingdom

1. Council of the British Medical Association, *War Crimes and Medicine* (Liverpool: Medical Education Trust, 1947).

2. *World Medical Association Bulletin* 1, no. 1 (1949): 3–14.

3. Peter Benenson, "The Forgotten Prisoners," *Guardian*, May 28, 1961, https:// www.theguardian.com/uk/1961/may/28/fromthearchive.theguardian.

4. Lord Parker of Waddington, *Report of the Committee of Privy Counsellors Appointed to Consider Authorised Procedures for the Interrogation of Persons Suspected of Terrorism*, March 1972, http://cain.ulst.ac.uk/hmso/parker.htm.

5. Kevin Boyle and Hurst Hannum, "Ireland in Strasbourg: Final Decisions in the Northern Irish Proceedings before the European Commission of Human Rights," *Irish Jurist* 11, no. 2 (Winter 1976): 243–78.

6. "British Government Authorised Use of Torture Methods in Northern Ireland in Early 1970s," BBC News, June 5, 2014, http://www.bbc.com/news/uk-northern -ireland-27714715; and Ireland v. the United Kingdom, no. 5310/71, European Court of Human Rights, Application, 5310/71, Strasberg, January 18, 1978, https://www.law.umich.edu/facultyhome/drwcasebook/Documents/Documents /Republic%20of%20Ireland%20v.%20United%20Kingdom.pdf.

7. "Governments Now Connive in Torture, Says Amnesty International," *Guardian*, December 12, 1972, https://www.theguardian.com/theguardian/2012/dec/12 /amnesty-anti-torture-campaign-1972.

8. Amnesty International, *Campaign for the Abolition of Torture*, ACT 40/004/1973, January 1, 1973, https://www.amnesty.org/en/documents/act40/004/1973/en/.

9. "The Doctor in Conflict," *British Medical Journal* 1, no. 5803 (March 25, 1972): 761–62, https://doi.org/10.1136/bmj.1.5803.761; and "The Doctor as Inquisitor," *Lancet* 299, no. 7753 (April 1, 1972): 732, https://doi.org/10.1016 /s0140–6736(72)90238–3.

10. Amnesty International, *Conference for the Abolition of Torture: Final Report*, ACT 40/002/1973 (London: Amnesty International, December 11, 1973).

11. UN General Assembly, Resolution 3452, Declaration on the Protection of All Persons from Being Subjected to Torture and Other Cruel, Inhuman or Degrading Treatment or Punishment (December 9, 1975), http://www.ohchr.org/EN /ProfessionalInterest/Pages/DeclarationTorture.aspx.

12. BMA, *Torture Report*.

13. BMA, *Medicine Betrayed*.

14. BMA, *The Medical Profession and Human Rights: Handbook for a Changing Agenda*. British Medical Association, London: Zed Books (in association with the BMA), 2001. [562 pp ISBN 1-85649-612-0 (p/b); 1-85649-611-2 (h/b); £50] https://www .amazon.com/Medical-Profession-Human-Rights-Handbook/dp/1856496120.

15. "BMA Procedures for Human Rights Interventions," BMA, 2009, accessed January 19, 2019, https://www.bma.org.uk/collective-voice/influence/international/global-justice/human-rights.

16. Salahadin Rastgeldi, *Aden Report*, MDE 27/002/1966 (London: Amnesty International, December 1966), https://www.amnesty.org/en/documents/mde27/002/1966/en/.

17. BMA, *Torture Report*.

18. Foreign and Commonwealth Office, Colonial Administration Files, April 24, 2014, https://www.gov.uk/guidance/colonial-administration-files.

19. European Center for Constitutional and Human Rights (ECCHR) and Public Interest Lawyers (PIL), *The Responsibility of Officials of the United Kingdom for War Crimes Involving Systematic Detainee Abuse in Iraq from 2003–2008* (Berlin: ECCHR, 2014).

20. REDRESS, "The Baha Mousa Case," accessed June 8, 2019, https://redress.org/casework/the-baha-mousa-case/; and Robert Fisk, "British Soldiers 'Kicked Iraqi Prisoner to Death,'" *Independent*, January 4, 2004, https://www.independent.co.uk/voices/commentators/fisk/british-soldiers-kicked-iraqi-prisoner-to-death-75721.html.

21. General Medical Council, *Fitness to Practice Panel of the Medical Practitioners Tribunal Service, Respondent Doctor: Dr. Derek Alexander Keilloh* (London: General Medical Council, December 2012).

22. General Medical Council, *Fitness to Practice Panel of the Medical Practitioners Tribunal Service, Respondent Doctor: Dr. Mohammed Al-Byati* (London: General Medical Council, March 3, 2014); "Iraqi Doctor 'Suspended over Torture Links,'" BBC News, March 1, 2013, https://www.bbc.com/news/uk-21633391.

23. "Vincent Bajinya," Trial International, June 6, 2018, https://trialinternational.org/latest-post/vincent-bajinya/; Athan Tashobya, "Genocide Suspects in UK Face Fresh Investigation," *New Times*, April 17, 2018, http://www.newtimes.co.rw/news/genocide-suspects-uk-face-fresh-investigation; and David Churchill, "Islington 'Genocide' Doctor Bailed by High Court Judge Who Raised Concern over Julian Assange–Style Asylum Bid," *Islington Gazette*, July 17, 2013, http://www.islingtongazette.co.uk/news/crime-courts/islington_genocide_doctor_bailed_by_high_court_judge_who_raised_concern_over_julian_assange_style_asylum_bid_1_2283861.

24. WMA, *WMA Statement on the Licensing of Physicians Fleeing Prosecution for Serious Criminal Offences*, November 1997, https://www.wma.net/policies-post/wma-statement-on-the-licensing-of-physicians-fleeing-prosecution-for-serious-criminal-offences/.

25. Graham Vanbergen, "Britain's Secret Widespread Use of Torture," *True Publica*, October 6, 2015, http://truepublica.org.uk/united-kingdom/britains-secret-widespread-use-torture/.

26. 736 Parl. Deb. (November 17, 1966) cols. 151–2W, in Corpun: World Corporal Punishment Research, http://www.corpun.com/ukpr6611.htm.

27. BMA, *Medical Profession and Human Rights*, 75.

28. UN Human Rights Office of the High Commissioner, Convention against Torture and Other Cruel, Inhuman or Degrading Treatment or Punishment (June 26, 1987), Article 14, https://www.ohchr.org/EN/ProfessionalInterest/Pages/CAT.aspx.

## Chapter 8. Humanists for Human Rights

1. Mary Ann Glendon, *A World Made New: Eleanor Roosevelt and the Universal Declaration of Human Rights* (New York: Random House, 2002); and Johannes Morsink, *The Universal Declaration of Human Rights: Origins, Drafting, and Intent* (Philadelphia: University of Pennsylvania Press, 1999).
2. William Korey, *NGOs and the Universal Declaration of Human Rights: A Curious Grapevine* (New York: Palgrave Macmillan, 2001).
3. UN General Assembly, Resolution 217A, Universal Declaration of Human Rights (December 10, 1948), http://www.un.org/en/universal-declaration-human-rights/index.html.
4. Korey, *NGOs and the Universal Declaration*; and Aryeh Neier, *The International Human Rights Movement: A History* (Princeton, NJ: Princeton University Press, 2013).
5. Neier, 78.
6. William A. Schabas, "Crime of Torture and the International Criminal Tribunals," *Case Western Reserve Journal of International Law* 37, no. 2 (2006): 349–64, https://scholarlycommons.law.case.edu/jil/vol37/iss2/11/.
7. Kathryn Sikkink, *The Justice Cascade: How Human Rights Prosecutions Are Changing World Politics* (New York: W. W. Norton, 2011); Juan E. Méndez and Marjory Wentworth, *Taking a Stand: The Evolution of Human Rights* (New York: Palgrave Macmillan, 2011); Priscilla B. Hayner, *Unspeakable Truths: Transitional Justice and the Challenge of Truth Commissions* (New York: Routledge, 2011); Samuel Moyn, *The Last Utopia: Human Rights in History* (Cambridge: Belknap Press, 2012).
8. Amnesty International, *Torture in Greece: The First Torturers' Trial 1975*, EUR 25/007/1977, April 1, 1977, https://www.amnesty.org/en/documents/eur25/007/1977/en/.
9. Stover and Nightingale, *Breaking of Bodies and Minds*, 33.
10. Lynn A. Hunt, *Inventing Human Rights: A History* (New York: W. W. Norton, 2007); Pinker, *Better Angels*, 587–90.
11. Matthijs Bal and Martijn Veltkamp, "How Does Fiction Reading Influence Empathy? An Experimental Investigation on the Role of Emotional Transportation," *PLOS*, January 30, 2013, https://doi.org/10.1371/journal.pone.0055341; and Joseph Frankel, "Reading Literature Won't Give You Superpowers," *Scientific American*, December 2, 2016.
12. Mark J. Harris, *Doctors of the Dark Side*, directed by Martha Davis (New York: Shelter Island Media, 2011).
13. Margaret Atwood, "Footnote to the Amnesty Report on Torture," in *Two-Headed Poems* (Oxford: Oxford University Press, 1978), 46; Carolyn Forché, "The Colonel," in *The Country between Us* (New York: Harper and Row, 1981), https://www.poetryfoundation.org/poems/49862/the-colonel; Harold Pinter, *One for the Road* (New York: Grove Weidenfeld, 1984).
14. John M. Coetzee, *Waiting for the Barbarians* (New York: Penguin Books, 1980), 5.
15. Mary W. Shelley, *Frankenstein* (New York: Dover Publications, 1994).
16. Robert L. Stevenson, *The Strange Case of Dr. Jekyll and Mr. Hyde* (North Miami Beach: Chump Change, 2017).

17. Herbert G. Wells, *The Island of Dr. Moreau* (New York: Bantam Classics, 1994).
18. Hans Janowitz and Carl Mayer, *The Cabinet of Dr. Caligari*, directed by Robert Wiene (1920; Potsdam: Decla-Bioscop AG, 1964).
19. Arthur Machen, *The Great God Pan* (London: Fantasy House, 1974); and Rosanne Rabinowitz, *Helen's Story* (Hornsea, UK: PS Publishing, 2013).
20. Friedrich Dürrenmatt, *Suspicion*, trans. Joel Agee (London: Pushkin Vertigo, 2017).
21. William Golding, *Free Fall* (New York: Mariner Books, 2003).
22. Ira Levin, *The Boys from Brazil* (New York: Pegasus Books, 2010).
23. Matthew Vaughn et al., *The Debt* (New York: Miramax, 2012).
24. Steve Sem-Sandberg, *The Chosen Ones: A Novel*, trans. Anna Patterson (New York: Farrar, Straus and Giroux, 2016).
25. Haruki Murakami, *Hard-Boiled Wonderland and the End of the World*, trans. Alfred Birnbaum (New York: Vintage International, 1993).
26. Shusaku Endo, *The Sea and Poison* (New York: New Directions, 1992), 166.
27. Andrey Iskanov, *Philosophy of a Knife*, directed by Andrey Iskanov (Russia: Unearthed Films, 2008).
28. George Orwell, *1984* (Fairfield, IA: First World Library, 2004), 304.
29. Anthony Burgess, *A Clockwork Orange* (New York: W. W. Norton, 1962), 95.
30. Burgess, 108.
31. Richard Condon, *The Manchurian Candidate* (New York: Pocket Star Books, 2004).
32. Valeriy Tarsis, *Ward 7: An Autobiographical Novel*, trans. Katya Brown (New York: E. P. Dutton, 1965).
33. Joseph A. Brodsky, "Gorbunov and Gorchakov," in *Collected Poems in English* (New York: Farrar, Straus and Giroux, 2000), 163.
34. Tom Stoppard, *Every Good Boy Deserves Favor and Professional Foul: Two Plays* (New York: Grove Press, 1994).
35. Aleksandr Solzhenitsyn, *A Day in the Life of Ivan Denisovitch*, trans. Harry T. Willetts (New York: Farrar, Straus and Giroux, 2005); and Aleksandr Solzhenitsyn, *The Gulag Archipelago: An Experiment in Literary Investigation* (New York: Harper and Row, 1973), 1:208, https://archive.org/details/TheGulagArchipelago -Threevolumes.
36. Vassilis Vassilikos, *Z* (New York: Pantheon Books, 1966).
37. Ariel Dorfman, *Death and the Maiden* (New York: Penguin Books, 1994).
38. Ariel Dorfman, "Death and the Maiden's Haunting Relevance: The Play I Wrote 20 Years Ago about Chile's Torture and Trauma Has a Painful, Global Relevance Today," *Guardian*, October 14, 2011, https://www.theguardian.com /commentisfree/2011/oct/14/death-maiden-relevance-play.
39. Michael Ondaatje, *Anil's Ghost* (London: Picador, 2001).
40. *Valley of the Wolves: Iraq*, directed by Serdar Akar and Sadullah Şentürk (Istanbul: Pana Films, 2007).
41. *Zero Dark Thirty*, directed by Kathryn Bigelow (Hollywood: Columbia Pictures, 2013); Michael Yudell, "The Problem with 'Zero Dark Thirty,'" *Inquirer Daily News*, February 22, 2013, http://www.philly.com/philly/blogs/public_health/The -problem-with-Zero-Dark-Thirty.html.
42. Edna O'Brien, *The Little Red Chairs* (New York: Back Bay Books, 2016).

43. "Sarajevo Red Line Project," *Remembering Srebrenica*, December 13, 2014, https:// www.srebrenica.org.uk/resources/research-resources/art-photography/sarajevo -red-line-project/.

44. Horace Engdahl, ed., *Witness Literature: Proceedings of the Nobel Centennial Symposium* (Stockholm: World Scientific Press, 2002), https://www.worldscientific.com /worldscibooks/10.1142/5103.

45. Lucette M. Lagnado and Sheila C. Dekel, *Children of the Flames: Dr. Josef Mengele and the Untold Story of the Twins of Auschwitz* (New York: Penguin Books, 1992).

46. Timerman, *Prisoner without a Name*, 54.

47. Susan Sontag, *Regarding the Pain of Others* (New York: Picador Press, 2004); and Michael Kimmelman, "Abu Ghraib Photos Return, This Time as Art," *New York Times*, October 10, 2004, https://www.nytimes.com/2004/10/10/arts/design/abu -ghraib-photos-return-this-time-as-art.html.

48. Steven Stanek, "Egyptian Bloggers Expose Horror of Police Torture," *SF Gate*, October 9, 2007, https://www.sfgate.com/politics/article/Egyptian-bloggers -expose-horror-of-police-torture-2536284.php; Jennifer Preston, "Movement Began with Outrage and a Facebook Page That Gave It an Outlet," *New York Times*, February 5, 2011, https://www.nytimes.com/2011/02/06/world/middleeast /06face.html; "Russian Authorities Probe Alleged Abuses in Prisons after Torture Video Emerges," Radio Free Europe, July 27, 2018, https://www.rferl.org /a/russian-authorities-probe-alleged-abuses-in-prisons-after-torture-video -emerges/29393969.html; and "Police 'Punished' as Torture Video Goes Viral," *The Nation*, January 26, 2019, https://nation.com.pk/26-Jan-2019/police-punished -as-torture-video-goes-viral.

49. Gadi Wolfsfeld, Elad Segev, and Tamir Sheafer, "Social Media and the Arab Spring: Politics Comes First," *International Journal of Press/Politics* 18, no. 2 (2013): 115– 37, https://journals.sagepub.com/doi/pdf/10.1177/1940161212471716.

## Chapter 9. Healers for Human Rights

1. Rejali, *Torture and Democracy*, 8–16.

2. Jonathon M. Mann, "Health and Human Rights," *British Medical Journal* 312, no. 7036 (April 1996): 924–25, https://www.ncbi.nlm.nih.gov/pmc/articles /PMC2350785; Jonathon M. Mann et al., "Health and Human Rights," *Health and Human Rights* 1, no. 1 (Fall 1994): 6–23, https://cdn2.sph.harvard.edu/wp -content/uploads/sites/13/2014/03/4-Mann.pdf; Michael A. Grodin et al., eds., *Health and Human Rights in a Changing World* (New York: Routledge, 2013); Amnesty International, *Prescription for Change: Health Professionals and the Exposure of Human Rights Violations*, ACT 75/001/1996, May 21, 1996, https://www .amnesty.org/en/documents/act75/001/1996/en/.

3. Korey, *NGOs and the Universal Declaration*, 423–42.

4. Tracy Ultveit-Moe, "The Story behind Our First Urgent Action, Forty Years Ago," *Amnesty International UK Urgent Action Network Blog*, March 19, 2013, https://www.amnesty.org.uk/blogs/urgent-action-network-blog/story-amnesty -first-ever-urgent-action-launched-forty-years-ago.

5. Amnesty International, *Amnesty International Health Professionals Network London Declaration*, ACT 75/005/1995, August 9, 1995, https://www.amnesty.org/en /documents/act75/005/1995/en/.

6. Amnesty International, *Doctors and Torture*, ACT 75/001/2002, March 1, 2002, https://www.amnesty.org/en/documents/act75/001/2002/en/; and Amnesty International, *Declaration on the Role of Health Professionals*.

7. Torsten Lucas and Christian Pross, "Caught between Conscience and Complicity: Human Rights Violations and the Health Professions," *Medicine and Global Survival* 2, no. 2 (June 1995): 106–14, http://www.ippnw.org/pdf/mgs/2–2-lucas .pdf.

8. Program for Torture Victims, "About Us," accessed June 8, 2019, http://ptvla.org /about-us/; "Our Founder," Helen Bamber Foundation: Working with Survivors of Human Cruelty, http://www.helenbamber.org/our-founder/.

9. International Rehabilitation Council for Torture Victims, http://www.irct.org/.

10. Center for Victims of Torture, http://www.cvt.org/.

11. Doug A. Johnson and Steven H. Miles, "As Full a Rehabilitation as Possible: Torture Survivors and the Right to Care," in *Realizing the Right to Health*, ed. Andrew Clapham and Mary Robinson (Zürich: Rüffer & Rub, 2009), 213–23.

12. WMA, *WMA Statement on the Right of Rehabilitation of Victims of Torture*, 2013, https://www.wma.net/policies-post/wma-statement-on-the-right-of -rehabilitation-of-victims-of-torture/.

13. Line Bager et al., "Does Multidisciplinary Rehabilitation of Tortured Refugees Represent 'Value-for-Money'? A Follow-up of a Danish Case-Study," *BMC Health Services Research* 18, no. 365 (May 18, 2018): 365–79, https://doi.org/10 .1186/s12913-018-3145-3.

14. Margaret Cunningham and Derrick Silove, "Principles of Treatment and Service Development for Torture and Trauma Survivors," in *International Handbook of Traumatic Stress Syndromes,* ed. John P. Wilson and Beverly Raphae (Boston: Springer, 1993), 751–62, https://doi.org/10.1007/978-1-4615-2820-3_63.

15. H. Vogel, F. Schmitz-Engels, and C. Grillo, "Radiology of Torture," *European Journal of Radiology* 63, no. 2 (August 2007): 187–204, https://doi.org/10.1016/j .ejrad.2007.03.036.

16. Lis Danielsen and Ole V. Rasmussen, "Dermatological Findings after Alleged Torture," *Torture* 16, no. 2 (February 2006): 108–27, https://doi.org/10.1016/j .forsciint.2014.08.037.

17. "Analytical Study about the Leaked Pictures of Torture Victims in Syrian Military Hospitals: 'The Photographed Holocaust,'" Syrian Network for Human Rights, October 15, 2015, http://sn4hr.org/blog/2015/10/15/12310/.

18. Stuart L. Lustig et al., "Asylum Grant Rates Following Medical Evaluations of Maltreatment among Political Asylum Applicants in the United States," *Journal of Immigrant and Minority Health* 10 (2008): 7–15.

19. James M. Jaranson and Michael K. Popkin, eds., *Caring for the Victims of Torture* (Washington, DC: American Psychiatric Press, 1998), 1–10.

20. "The Amnesty Human Rights Award 2018 Goes to the Nadeem Centre for Its Fight against Torture in Egypt," Amnesty International, January 24, 2018, https://

www.amnesty.de/informieren/artikel/aegypten-amnesty-human-rights-award
-2018-goes-nadeem-centre-its-fight-against-0.

21. Neier, *International Human Rights Movement*, 258–84.
22. Kelly N. Owens, Michelle Harvey-Blankenship, and Mary-Claire King, "Genomic Sequencing in the Service of Human Rights," *International Journal of Epidemiology* 31, no. 1 (February 2002): 53–58, https://doi.org/10.1093/ije/31.1.53.
23. Korey, *NGOs and the Universal Declaration*, 427.
24. Stephen G. Michaud, "Identifying Argentina's Disappeared," *New York Times Magazine*, December 27, 1987, https://www.nytimes.com/1987/12/27/magazine /identifying-argentina-s-disappeared.html.
25. Neil J. Kritz, *Transitional Justice: How Emerging Democracies Reckon with Former Regimes* (Washington, DC: US Institute of Peace Press, 1995), 279; Margaret Cox et al., eds., *The Scientific Investigation of Mass Graves: Towards Protocols and Standard Operating Procedures* (Cambridge: Cambridge University Press, 2014).
26. Andrew A. Skolnick, "Bearing Witness for the Dead," *Medhunters*, Winter 2001, 14–17, http://www.aaskolnick.com/new/articles/Medhunters.pdf.
27. Clea Koff, *The Bone Woman: A Forensic Anthropologist's Search for Truth in the Mass Graves of Rwanda, Bosnia, Croatia, and Kosovo* (New York: Random House, 2005).
28. "Worldwide Appeals," *Amnesty International Newsletter*, December 1993, 1, https://www.amnesty.org/download/Documents/184000/nws210091993en.pdf.
29. Vincent Iacopino, "Turkish Physicians Coerced to Conceal Systematic Torture," *Lancet* 348, no. 9040 (November 1996): 1500, https://doi.org/10.1016/S0140–6736(05)65892–8; Vincent Iacopino et al., "Physician Complicity in Misrepresentation and Omission of Evidence of Torture in Post-Detention Medical Examinations in Turkey," *JAMA* 276, no. 5 (September 1996): 396–402, https://jamanetwork.com/journals/jama/article-abstract/406048.
30. David S. Weissbrodt, "International Measures against Arbitrary Killings by Governments," *American Society of International Law* 77 (1983): 378–404, https://www.cambridge.org/core/journals/proceedings-of-the-asil-annual-meeting /article/international-measures-against-arbitrary-killings-by-governments /BC5D053ED37A7F5B55E9A2B6BCCA3A65.
31. UN Department of Political Affairs, *United Nations Manual on the Effective Prevention and Investigation of Extra-Legal, Arbitrary, and Summary Executions*, E/ST/CSDHA/ (1991), 12, https://www.un.org/ruleoflaw/files/UN_Manual_on _the_Effective_Prevention_and_Investigation%5B1%5D.pdf; David S. Weissbrodt and Terri Rosen, "Principles against Executions," *Hamline Law Review* 13 (1990): 579–623; and UN Human Rights Office of the High Commissioner, *The Minnesota Protocol on the Investigation of Potentially Unlawful Death (2016): The Revised United Nations Manual on the Effective Prevention and Investigation of Extra-legal, Arbitrary, and Summary Executions* (New York: United Nations Publications, 2017), 1–87, https://www.ohchr.org/Documents/Publications /MinnesotaProtocol.pdf.
32. Ruben Rosario, "Justice Achieved in Guatemala, Thanks to the Minnesota Protocol," *Pioneer Press*, May 16, 2013, https://www.twincities.com/2013/05/15/ruben -rosario-justice-achieved-in-guatemala-thanks-to-the-minnesota-protocol/.

33. Vincent Iacopino, Onder Ozkalipci, and Caroline Schlar, "The Istanbul Protocol: International Standards for the Effective Investigation and Documentation of Torture and Ill Treatment," *Lancet* 354, no. 9184 (September 25, 1999): 1117, https://doi.org/10.1016/s0140-6736(99)08381-6; Helen McColl, Kamaldeep Bhui, and Edgar Jones, "The Role of Doctors in Investigation, Prevention, and Treatment of Torture," *Journal of the Royal Society of Medicine* 105, no. 11 (November 2012): 464–71, https://doi.org/10.1258/jrsm.2012.120100.

34. Office of the UN High Commissioner for Human Rights, *Istanbul Protocol: Manual on the Effective Investigation and Documentation of Torture and Other Cruel, Inhuman or Degrading Treatment or Punishment*, HR/P/PT/8/Rev.1 (August 9, 1999), https://www.ohchr.org/documents/publications/training8rev1en.pdf.

35. PHR, *Istanbul Protocol Model Medical Curriculum: Model Curriculum on the Effective Medical Documentation of Torture and Ill-Treatment*, 2006–9, http://phrtoolkits.org/toolkits/istanbul-protocol-model-medical-curriculum/; "IRCT Awarded EC Grant for Follow-Up of the Istanbul Protocol Implementation Project (IPIP)," IRCT, September 14, 2005, https://irct.org/media-and-resources/latest-news/article/180.

36. WMA, *Resolution on the Responsibility of Physicians in the Documentation and Denunciation of Acts of Torture or Cruel or Inhuman or Degrading Treatment*, September 2003, amended October 2007, https://www.wma.net/policies-post/wma-resolution-on-the-responsibility-of-physicians-in-the-documentation-and-denunciation-of-acts-of-torture-or-cruel-or-inhuman-or-degrading-treatment/.

37. Mark Bollman et al., "Investigation of Deaths in Custody," in *Monitoring Detention, Custody, Torture and Ill-Treatment: A Practical Approach to Prevention and Documentation*, ed. Jason Payne-James, Jonathan Beynon, and Duarte N. Vieira (Boca Raton, FL: CRC Press, 2018), 241–45.

38. International Forensic Expert Group, "Statement on Access to Relevant Medical and Other Health Records and Relevant Legal Records for Forensic Medical Evaluations of Alleged Torture and Other Cruel, Inhuman or Degrading Treatment or Punishment," *Journal of Forensic and Legal Medicine* 20, no. 3 (April 2013): 158–63.

39. Human Rights Watch, *"It's Part of the Job": Ill-Treatment and Torture of Vulnerable Groups in Lebanese Police Stations*, June 26, 2013, https://www.hrw.org/report/2013/06/26/its-part-job/Ill-Treatment-and-torture-vulnerable-groups-lebanese-police-stations.

40. "Alleged Police Torture: PHC Cancels Doctor's Transfer Orders," *Express Tribune*, October 11, 2012, https://tribune.com.pk/story/449889/alleged-police-torture-phc-cancels-doctors-transfer-orders/.

41. Al Nadeem Center for Rehabilitation of Victims of Violence, *Joint HR Statement in Solidarity with Egyptian Doctors Protesting Police Brutality*, February 11, 2016, https://www.alnadeem.org/en/content/joint-hr-statement-solidarity-egyptian-doctors-protesting-police-brutality; "Egypt Shuts El Nadeem Centre for Torture Victims," *Al Jazeera News*, February 9, 2017, https://www.aljazeera.com/news/2017/02/egypt-shuts-el-nadeem-centre-torture-victims-170209143119775.html.

42. Germaine DeLarch, "Kenya Medical Association Issues Statement on Forced Examinations," *Pan Africa ILGA*, September 28, 2017, http://panafricailga.org

/breaking-kenya-medical-association-issues-statement-on-forced-examinations/; Nita Bhalla, "Rare Win for Gay Rights as Kenya Court Rules Forced Anal Tests Illegal," Reuters, March 22, 2018, https://af.reuters.com/article/africaTech /idAFL3N1R45E4.

43. "Tunisia: Doctors Oppose 'Anal Test' for Homosexuality," Human Rights Watch, April 12, 2017, https://www.hrw.org/news/2017/04/12/tunisia-doctors-oppose -anal-test-homosexuality; AFP, "Tunisia to End 'Inhuman' Forced Anal Examinations on 'Suspected Homosexuals,'" TheJournal.ie, September 23, 2017, http:// www.thejournal.ie/tunisia-anal-exams-3611526-Sep2017/.

44. Amnesty International, *Amnesty International Annual Report 2016–2017*, 2017, 190, https://www.amnesty.org/en/latest/research/2017/02/amnesty-international -annual-report-201617/.

45. Michael Cook, "Israeli Doctors Refuse to Feed Hunger-Striker," *BioEdge*, August 16, 2015, https://www.bioedge.org/bioethics/israeli-doctors-refuse-to -feed-hunger-striker/11528#.Vc9b4Jf7Fus.facebook.

46. Open Society Initiative for Southern Africa, Open Society Institute, and Bellevue/ NYU Program for Survivors of Torture, *"We Have Degrees in Violence": A Report on Torture and Human Rights Abuses in Zimbabwe*, December 2007, https://www .opensocietyfoundations.org/publications/we-have-degrees-violence-report -torture-and-human-rights-abuses-zimbabwe.

47. Ruth Michaelson, "Egypt's Nadeem Center for Torture Victims Persists against Odds," *Deutsche Welle*, April 16, 2018, https://www.dw.com/en/egypts-nadeem -center-for-torture-victims-persists-against-odds/a-43388534.

48. Godfrey Ssali, "Kaweesi Murder Suspects to Get Sh80 Million Compensation," *Independent*, October 13, 2017, https://www.independent.co.ug/tortured-kaweesi -murder-suspects-get-80-million-shillings/.

49. Joshua Colangelo-Bryan and Joe Stork, *Torture Redux: The Revival of Physical Coercion during Interrogations in Bahrain* (New York: Human Rights Watch, February 8, 2010), http://www.hrw.org/reports/2010/02/08/torture-redux-0; UK Home Office, *Report of Fact-Finding Mission to Cameroon, 17–25 January 2004*, January 25, 2004, http://www.refworld.org/docid/4152c6cc4.html; Open Society Initiative for Southern Africa et al., *"We Have Degrees in Violence."*

50. "Sudan's Doctors Union Says 57 Killed in Recent Protests," Associated Press, February 8, 2019, https://www.apnews.com/5775125fac91424594f74fc099b 9a642.

51. Eliza Munoz, "Patient-Physician Confidentiality on Trial in Turkey," *JAMA* 276, no. 17 (1996): 1375–76, https://doi.org/10.1001/jama.1996.03540170019011.

52. AAAS Science and Human Rights Program, "Physician Charged in Turkey," AAAS Human Rights Action Network Alert, May 12, 1997.

53. Clive S. Lewis, *The Screwtape Letters* (New York: MacMillian, 1968), 137.

## Chapter 10. Organized Medicine's Condemn and Abide

1. WMA, "Who Can Be a WMA Member?," https://www.wma.net/who-we-are /members/.

2. WMA, "Torture Prevention," https://www.wma.net/what-we-do/human-rights /torture-prevention/.

3. Steven H. Miles and Alfred M. Freedman, "Medical Ethics and Torture: Revising the Declaration of Tokyo," *Lancet* 373, no. 9660 (January 2009): 344–48, https:// doi.org/10.1016/s0140–6736(09)60097–0.

4. Miles and Freedman.

5. WMA, *International Code of Medical Ethics*, October 1949, https://www.wma.net /policies-post/wma-international-code-of-medical-ethics/international-code-of -medical-ethics-2006/.

6. International Committee of the Red Cross (ICRC), *Geneva Convention Relative to the Treatment of Prisoners of War (Third Geneva Convention)*, 1949, https://www .refworld.org/docid/3ae6b36c8.html.

7. UN Economic and Social Council, Resolution 663C, Standard Minimum Rules for the Treatment of Prisoners (July 31, 1957), https://www.unodc.org /pdf/criminal_justice/UN_Standard_Minimum_Rules_for_the_Treatment_of _Prisoners.pdf/.

8. WMA, *Regulations in Times of Armed Conflict and Other Situations of Violence*, October 1956, https://www.wma.net/policies-post/wma-regulations-in-times-of -armed-conflict-and-other-situations-of-violence/.

9. Amnesty International, *Conference for the Abolition of Torture: Paris December 10–11 1973: Final Report*, 1973, 1–32, https://www.amnesty.org/en/documents/act40/002 /1973/en/.

10. WMA, *Declaration of Tokyo*.

11. UN General Assembly, Principles of Medical Ethics, A/RES/37/194 (December 18, 1982), http://www.un.org/documents/ga/res/37/a37r194.htm.

12. UN General Assembly, Convention against Torture and Other Cruel, Inhuman or Degrading Treatment or Punishment, A/RES/39/46 (December 10, 1984), http:// www.un.org/documents/ga/res/39/a39r046.htm.

13. UN General Assembly, Body of Principles for the Protection of All Persons under Any Form of Detention or Imprisonment, A/RES/43/173 (December 9, 1988), http://www.un.org/documents/ga/res/43/a43r173.htm.

14. Rome Statute of the International Criminal Court, A/CONF.183/9, July 17, 1998, https://www.icc-cpi.int/nr/rdonlyres/ea9aeff7-5752-4f84-be94–0a655eb30e16/0 /rome_statute_english.pdf.

15. John R. Bolton, "International Criminal Court: Letter to UN Secretary General Kofi Annan," US Department of State, May 6, 2002, https://2001–2009.state.gov /r/pa/prs/ps/2002/9968.htm.

16. Diane M. Amann and Mortimer N. S. Sellers, "The United States of America and the International Criminal Court," University of Georgia School of Law, January 1, 2002, http://digitalcommons.law.uga.edu/fac_artchop/670/; Kip Hale, "Why the U.S. Can No Longer Ignore the ICC," *Foreign Affairs*, November 16, 2017, https://www.foreignaffairs.com/articles/afghanistan/2017-11-16/why-us-can-no -longer-ignore-icc.

17. Yasemin N. Oguz and Steven H. Miles, "The Physician and Prison Hunger Strikes: Reflecting on the Experience in Turkey," *Journal of Medical Ethics* 31, no.

3 (February 2005): 169–72, https://doi.org/10.1136/jme.2004.006973; Padraig O'Malley, *Biting at the Grave: The Irish Hunger Strikes and the Politics of Despair* (Boston: Beacon Press, 1990); and Steven Erlanger, "Palestinians on Fast in Israeli Jails Struggle for Attention," *New York Times*, August 28, 2004, https://www .nytimes.com/2004/08/28/world/palestinians-on-fast-in-israeli-jails-struggle-for -attention.html.

18. UN Office of the High Commissioner for Human Rights, "IACHR, UN Working Group on Arbitrary Detention, UN Rapporteur on Torture, UN Rapporteur on Human Rights and Counter-Terrorism, and UN Rapporteur on Health Reiterate Need to End the Indefinite Detention of Individuals at Guantanamo Naval Base in Light of Current Human Rights Crisis," news release, May 1, 2013, https:// newsarchive.ohchr.org/AR/NewsEvents/Pages/DisplayNews.aspx?NewsID= 13278&LangID=E; ICRC, *Hunger Strikes in Prisons: The ICRC's Position*, January 31, 2013, https://www.icrc.org/en/document/hunger-strikes-prisons-icrc-position; and Hernán Reyes, "Medical and Ethical Aspects of Hunger Strikes in Custody and the Issue of Torture," ICRC, January 1, 1998, https://www.icrc.org/eng/resources /documents/article/other/health-article-010198.htm.

19. WMA, *Declaration of Malta on Hunger Strikers*, November 1991, https://www .wma.net/policies-post/wma-declaration-of-malta-on-hunger-strikers/; PHR, "Hunger Strikes and the Practice of Force-Feeding," October 2013, http:// physiciansforhumanrights.org/library/other/hunger-strikes-and-the-practice-of -force-feeding.html.

20. Juan O. Tamayo, "Cuban Dissident Rejects Offer, Continues Hunger Strike," *Human Rights in Cuba* (blog), November 9, 2013, https://humanrightsincuba .blogspot.com/2013/11/cuban-dissident-rejects-offer-continues.html; "India Must Release Prisoner of Conscience on Prolonged Hunger Strike," Amnesty International India, October 1, 2013, https://amnesty.org.in/news-update/india -must-release-prisoner-conscience-prolonged-hunger-strike/; WMA, "WMA Warned about Mounting Campaign against Turkish Doctors," January 2, 2001, https://www.wma.net/news-post/wma-warned-about-mounting-campaign -against-turkish-doctors/; George J. Annas, Sondra S. Crosby, and Leonard H. Glantz, "Guantanamo Bay: A Medical Ethics-Free Zone?," *New England Journal of Medicine* 369, no. 2 (July 2013): 101–3, https://doi.org/10.1056/nejmp1306065.

21. "Charles Twagira," Trial International, February 14, 2018, https://trialinternational .org/latest-post/charles-twagira/.

22. "Eugene Rwamucyo," Trial International, June 1, 2016, https://trialinternational .org/latest-post/eugene-rwamucyo/.

23. David Churchill, "Islington 'Genocide' Doctor Bailed by High Court Judge Who Raised Concern over Julian Assange–Style Asylum Bid," *Islington Gazette*, July 17, 2013, http://www.islingtongazette.co.uk/news/crime-court/islington -genocide-doctor-bailed-by-high-court-judge-who-raised-concern-over-julian -assange-style-asylum-bid-1-2283861.

24. WMA, *Resolution on the Responsibility of Physicians*.

25. WMA, *Declaration of Tokyo*.

26. WMA, *Resolution on Prohibition of Forced*.

27. World Psychiatric Association (WPA), *Madrid Declaration on Ethical Standards for Psychiatric Practice*, August 25, 1996, http://www.wpanet.org/detail.php?section _id=5&content_id=48.

28. WPA, "Declaration on Participation of Psychiatrists in Interrogation of Detainees," *Torture* 27, no. 3 (October 2017): 96–98, https://doi.org/10.7146/torture .v27i3.103980.

29. Sharon Shalev, "Solitary Confinement: The View from Europe," *Canadian Journal of Human Rights* 4, no. 1 (November 18, 2015), https://ssrn.com/abstract= 3073611.

30. Peter Scharff Smith, "The Effects of Solitary Confinement on Prison Inmates: A Brief History and Review of the Literature," *Crime and Justice* 34 (2006): 441– 528; and Craig Haney, "The Psychological Effects of Solitary Confinement: A Systematic Critique," *Crime and Justice* 47, no. 1 (March 2018): 365–416, https:// www.journals.uchicago.edu/doi/abs/10.1086/696041.

31. International Psychological Trauma Symposium, "The Istanbul Statement on the Use and Effects of Solitary Confinement," *Torture* 16, no. 1 (2008): 63–66, https:// irct.org/assets/uploads/Opinion.pdf.

32. UN General Assembly, Torture and Other Cruel, Inhuman or Degrading Treatment or Punishment [note], A/63/175 (July 28, 2008), 18–21, https://documents -dds-ny.un.org/doc/UNDOC/GEN/N08/440/75/PDF/N0844075.pdf.

33. Amnesty International, *Entombed: Isolation in the US Federal Prison System*, July 16, 2014, https://www.amnestyusa.org/reports/entombed-isolation-in-the-us-federal -prison-system/; Samy Magdy, "Rights Group: Egypt Uses Solitary Confinement as 'Torture,'" Associated Press, May 7, 2018, https://www.apnews.com /5372a8e0b4534cd2a09c63d539ed6f09; Christy Carnegie Fujio and Mike Corradin, *Buried Alive: Solitary Confinement in the US Detention System* (New York: PHR, 2013), http://physiciansforhumanrights.org/library/reports/buried-alive-solitary -confinement-in-the-us-detention-system.html; and Sharon Shalev, *A Sourcebook on Solitary Confinement* (Oxford: Center for Criminology, Oxford University, 2008), http://eprints.lse.ac.uk/24557/1/SolitaryConfinementSourcebookPrint.pdf.

34. United Nations, "Standard Minimum Rules on the Treatment of Prisons" (Mandela Rules), 2015, http://solitaryconfinement.org/mandela-rules.

35. UN General Assembly, Resolution 37/194, Principles of Medical Ethics Relevant to the Role of Health Personnel, Particularly Physicians, in the Protection of Prisoners and Detainees against Torture and Other Cruel, Inhuman or Degrading Treatment or Punishment (December 18, 1982), http://www.un.org/documents /ga/res/37/a37r194.htm.

36. WMA, *Statement on Solitary Confinement*, 2014, https://www.wma.net/policies -post/wma-statement-on-solitary-confinement/.

37. Andrew Cohen, "Death, Yes, but Torture at Supermax?," *Atlantic Monthly*, June 4, 2012, https://www.theatlantic.com/national/archive/2012/06/death-yes-but-torture -at-supermax/258002/; Laurel Wamsley, "September 11 Conspirator Files Lawsuit Saying His Isolation Is 'Psychological Torture,'" National Public Radio, February 6, 2018, https://www.npr.org/sections/thetwo-way/2018/02/06/583714408/sept-11 -conspirator-files-lawsuit-saying-his-isolation-is-psychological-torture; and Angela

Browne, Alissa Cambier, and Suzanne Agha, "Prisons within Prisons: The Use of Segregation in the United States," *Federal Sentencing Reporter* 24, no. 1 (October 2011): 46–49, https://doi.org/10.1525/fsr.2011.24.1.46.

38. Cyrus Ahaltr, Alex Rothman, and Brie A. Williams, "Examining the Role of Healthcare Professionals in the Use of Solitary Confinement," *British Medical Journal* 359 (October 2017): 4657, https://doi.org/ 10.1136/bmj.j4657.

39. CPT, *Report to the Croatian Government*, CPT/Inf (2014) 9, 24.

40. WMA, *Resolution Supporting the Rights of Patients and Physicians in the Islamic Republic of Iran*, 2009, https://www.wma.net/policies-post/wma-resolution -supporting-the-rights-of-patients-and-physicians-in-the-islamic-republic-of -iran/; "159th Council Meeting," WMA, May 8, 2001, https://www.wma.net/news -post/world-medical-association-159th-council-meeting/.

41. WMA, *Resolution on Health and Human Rights Abuses in Zimbabwe*, October 2007, https://www.wma.net/policies-post/wma-resolution-on-health-and-human-rights -abuses-in-zimbabwe/.

42. "WMA Condemns Use of Doctors in Saudi Arabia Flogging," WMA, February 5, 2015, https://www.wma.net/news-post/wma-condemns-use-of-doctors-in -saudi-arabia-flogging/.

43. "WMA Urges Immediate Release of Surgeon Jailed in Egypt," WMA, January 18, 2016, https://www.wma.net/news-post/wma-urges-immediate-release-of-surgeon -jailed-in-egypt/.

44. WMA, *Declaration of Hamburg concerning Support for Medical Doctors Refusing to Participate in, or to Condone, the Use of Torture and Other Cruel, Inhuman or Degrading Treatment*, November 1997, https://www.wma.net/policies-post/wma -declaration-of-hamburg-concerning-support-for-medical-doctors-refusing-to -participate-in-or-to-condone-the-use-of-torture-or-other-forms-of-cruel -inhuman-or-degrading-treatment/.

45. WMA, *WMA Council Resolution on Prohibition of Physician Participation in Torture*, May 2009, https://www.wma.net/policies-post/wma-council-resolution-on -prohibition-of-physician-participation-in-torture/.

46. WMA, *Recommendation on the Development of a Monitoring and Reporting Mechanism to Permit Audit of Adherence of States to the Declaration of Tokyo*, October 2011, https://www.wma.net/policies-post/wma-recommendation-on-the-development -of-a-monitoring-and-reporting-mechanism-to-permit-audit-of-adherence-of -states-to-the-declaration-of-tokyo/.

47. BMA, *Medical Profession and Human Rights*, 420.

## Chapter 11: Innovations

1. Neil J. Kritz, *Transitional Justice: How Emerging Democracies Reckon with Former Regimes* (Washington, DC: US Institute of Peace Press, 1995), 279; Amnesty International, *Torture in Greece*.

2. Stover and Nightingale, *Breaking of Bodies and Minds*, 33.

3. Don H. Foster and Dennis Davis, *Detention and Torture in South Africa, Psychological, Legal and Historical Studies* (New York: St. Martin's Press, 1987); Laurel

Baldwin-Ragaven, Jeanelle De Gruchy, and Leslie London, *An Ambulance of the Wrong Colour: Health Professionals, Human Rights and Ethics in South Africa* (Ndabeni: University of Cape Town Press, 1999).

4. "Truth Commission Special Report Transcript: Episode 1, Section 10," South African Broadcasting Company, accessed June 9, 2019, http://sabctrc.saha.org.za /tvseries/episode1/section10.htm.

5. Tony Karon, "Remembering the Death of Steve Biko 35 Years Later," *Time*, September 12, 2012, http://time.com/3791503/remembering-the-death-of-steve -biko-35-years-later/.

6. Winfried Beck, "The World Medical Association Serves Apartheid," *International Journal of Health Services* 20, no. 1 (January 1990): 185–91.

7. Mandisa Mbali, "'A Matter of Conscience': The Moral Authority of the World Medical Association and the Readmission of the South Africans, 1976–1994," *Medical History* 58, no. 2 (April 28, 2014): 257–77, https://doi.org/10.1017/mdh .2014.8.

8. Lawrence Baxter, "Doctors on Trial: Steve Biko, Medical Ethics, and the Courts," *South African Journal on Human Rights* 1 (January 1985): 137–51, https://scholarship .law.duke.edu/cgi/viewcontent.cgi?article=2678&context=faculty_scholarship; Charles H. Wright, "Opposition to the World Medical Association Assembly in South Africa, 1985," *Journal of the National Medical Association* 77, no. 7 (July 1985): 541–42, https://www.ncbi.nlm.nih.gov/pmc/articles/PMC2571134/.

9. "NAMDA–National Medical and Dental Association," South African History Online, August 1989, 30–32, http://www.sahistory.org.za/archive/namda-national -medical-and-dental-association.

10. "A Brief History of the National Medical and Dental Association (NAMDA)," *Critical Health*, 25 (December 1988): 58–66, http://www.sahistory.org.za/archive /a-brief-history-of-the-national-medical-and-dental-association-%28namda%29.

11. Graeme R. Mclean and Trefor Jenkins, "The Steve Biko Affair: A Case Study in Medical Ethics," *Developing World Bioethics* 3, no. 1 (2003): 77–95, https://doi.org /10.1111/1471–8847.00060; Sheila Rule, "Pretoria Doctor Loses His License," *New York Times*, October 17, 1985, https://www.nytimes.com/1985/10/17/world /pretoria-doctor-loses-his-license.html.

12. "The Apartheid Government Reportedly Pays Compensation for Death of Steve Biko," South African History Online, July 29, 1979, http://www.sahistory.org.za /dated-event/apartheid-government-reportedly-pays-compensation-death-steve -biko.

13. Nosipiwo Manona and Nicki Gules, "The Grim Legacy of Steve Biko's Killer," *City Press*, September 17, 2017, https://www.news24.com/SouthAfrica/News/the -grim-legacy-of-steve-bikos-killer-20170917-2.

14. Bernard B. Mandell, G. P. Damster, and H. A. Hanekom, "MASA [Medical Association of South Africa] and a Truth Commission for the Medical Profession," *South African Medical Journal* 86, no. 9 (1996): 1070–71, https://repository.library .georgetown.edu/handle/10822/896269.

15. "New Medical Association Starts in South Africa," *British Medical Journal* 317, no. 7152 (July 1998): 166, https://doi.org/10.1136/bmj.317.7152.166b.

16. Tarsis, *Ward 7*.
17. Sidney Bloch and Peter Reddaway, *Soviet Psychiatric Abuse: The Shadow over World Psychiatry* (London: Victor Gollancz, 1984); Walter Reich, "The World of Soviet Psychiatry," *New York Times*, January 30, 1983, https://www.nytimes.com /1983/01/30/magazine/the-world-of-soviet-psychiatry.html; Stover and Nightingale, *Breaking of Bodies and Minds*, 129–252; Carl Gershman, "Psychiatric Abuse in the Soviet Union," *Society* 21, no. 5 (1984): 54–59, https://doi.org/10.1007 /BF02695434; Bloch and Reddaway, *Russia's Political Hospitals*.
18. Koryagin, "Unwilling Patients."
19. Peter B. Reddaway, "The Attack on Anatoly Koryagin," *New York Review of Books*, March 3, 1983, https://www.nybooks.com/articles/1983/03/03/the-attack-on -anatoly-koryagin/; Koryagin, "Involvement of Soviet Psychiatry," 336–40.
20. Vera Rich, "Soviet Psychiatry: Pre-Emptive Resignation?," *Nature* 301, no. 5901 (February 1983): 559, https://doi.org/10.1038/301559a0.
21. J. Patrice McSherry, *Predatory States: Operation Condor and Covert War in Latin America* (Lanham, MD: Rowman and Littlefield, 2005).
22. Maxwell G. Bloche, "Uruguay's Military Physicians: Cogs in a System of State Terror," *JAMA* 255, no. 20 (1986): 2788–93, https://doi.org/10.1001/jama.1986 .03370200090034; and "Uruguay: Los Médicos Cómplices de la Dictadura Militar" [Uruguay: The medical accomplices of the military dictatorship], *Viejo Blues*, June 5, 2008.
23. Inter-American Commission on Human Rights, *Resolution No. 11/84, Case No. 9274: Uruguay*, October 3, 1984, http://www.cidh.org/annualrep/84.85eng /Uruguay9274.htm; and Gregorio Martirena, "Fuimos los primeros en enjuiciar a un médico por torturas" [We were the first to prosecute a doctor for torture], *Noticias* (Sindicato Médico del Uruguay), 1984, accessed July 30, 2018, http:// www.smu.org.uy/publicaciones/noticias/separ99/art6.htm.
24. Gregorio Martirena, "The Medical Profession and Torture," *Journal of Medical Ethics* 17 (December 1991): S23–25, https://doi.org/10.1136/jme.17.Suppl.23; Richard Goldstein and Alfred Gellhorn, *Human Rights and the Medical Profession in Uruguay since 1972* (Washington, DC: American Association for the Advancement of Science, 1982), https://www.ncbi.nlm.nih.gov/nlmcatalog/100944931; Amando Olivera, interview with Gregario Martirena, SMU, archived March 7, 2009, https://www .smu.org.uy/publicaciones/noticias/separ99/art6.htm; "Uruguay: Acusan Medico Complice Toruras," *Clarín*, February 13, 1999, https://www.clarin.com/ediciones -anteriores/uruguay-acusan-medico-complice-torturas_0_BkBWhrRl0Fx.html; "Fallo del consejo arbitral del SMU respecto de la dra. Rosa Marsicano" [Decision of the arbitration council of the SMU regarding Dr. Rosa Marsicano], *Noticias* (Sindicato Médico del Uruguay), February 21, 2000, http://www.smu.org.uy /publicaciones/noticias/noticias103/art10.htm; Gregorio Martirena, "Uruguay: Torture and Doctors," *Torture* S2 (1992); "Expulsión de FEMI: Doctor Juan Antonio Riva Buglio" [Expulsion from FEMI: Doctor Juan Antonio Riva Buglio], *Memoria Viva* (blog), October 7, 2008, http://memoriaviva5.blogspot.com/2008/07 /expulsin-de-femi-doctor-juan-antonio.html; "El-SMU Expulso-a-Medica-Militar-por-su-Actuacion-Durante-la-Dictadura," *La Republica*, February 29, 2000;

"Doctors, Ethics and Torture," *Danish Medical Bulletin* 34, no. 4 (August 1987): 185–216; Martirena, "Fuimos los primeros"; Lucas and Pross, "Caught between Conscience," 106–13; Mary Yics, "Uruguay: Opinion and Human Rights," *Gacetillas Argentinas* (blog), June 3, 2008, http://gacetillasargentinas.blogspot.com/2008 /06/newsletter-internacionales-040608_4.html; and "SUMA: Denuncia penal crímenes de lesa humanidad," Observatorio Luz Ibarburu, accessed July 30, 2018, http://www.observatorioluzibarburu.org/media/uploads/1774482011.pdf.

25. Rosario Touriño, "Médicos involucrados en violaciones de derechos humanos siguen en actividad" [Doctors involved in human rights violations are still active], *Agaton* (blog), May 22, 2014, https://carlosagaton.blogspot.com/2014/05/medicos-involucrados-en-violaciones-de.html.

26. "Conheça e acesse o relatório final da CNV" [Get to know and access the CNV final report], Comissão Nacional de Verdade [National Truth Commission], December 10, 2014, http://cnv.memoriasreveladas.gov.br/index.php/outros -destaques/574-conheca-e-acesse-o-relatorio-final-da-cnv.

27. Amnesty International, *Brazil: Human Rights Violations and the Health Professions*, AMR 19/025/1996, October 11, 1996, https://www.amnesty.org/en/documents /amr19/025/1996/en/; and Pedro Venceslau, "A verdade sobre os médicos da ditadura" [The truth about the doctors of the dictatorship], *Forum*, June 27, 2012, https://www.revistaforum.com.br/a-verdade-sobre-os-medicos-da-ditadura/.

28. Paulo E. Arns, *Brasil, Nunca Mais* [Brazil, never again] (Petrópolis: Vozes, 1985); Archdiocese of São Paulo, *Torture in Brazil: A Shocking Report on the Pervasive Use of Torture by Brazilian Military Governments, 1964–1979*, ed. Joan Dassin, trans. Jaime Wright (Austin: University of Texas Press, 1998).

29. Conselho Regional de Medicina de São Paulo [Regional Council of Medicine of São Paulo], "Questão de justiça" [Question of justice], October–December 2008, 18, http://www.cremesp.com.br/?siteAcao=Revista&id=388.

30. Aureliano Biancarelli, "Os médicos e a ditadura militar" [The doctors and the military dictatorship], Counselho Regional de Medicina do Estado de São Paulo, July–September 2015, 16–29, http://www.cremesp.org.br/?siteAcao=Revista&id=803.

31. Summer Volkmer, "Sanctions for Torture: Domestic Medical Associations Take Action," *Berkeley Law*, June 2010, https://www.law.berkeley.edu/experiential /clinics/international-human-rights-law-clinic/do-no-harm-intelligence-ethics -health-professionals-and-the-torture-debate/sanctions-by-medical-associations -for-torture/.

32. Amnesty International, *Prescription for Change: Health Professionals and the Exposure of Human Rights Violations*, ACT 75/001/1996, May 21, 1996, https://www .amnesty.org/en/documents/act75/001/1996/en/.

33. "Médicos Legistas Negam Fraudes em Laudos de Militantes en Ditadura" [Medical doctors deny fraud in reports during military dictatorship], *Globo* (Rio de Janeiro), July 5, 2015, http://g1.globo.com/rio-de-janeiro/noticia/2015/05/medicos -legistas-negam-fraudes-em-laudos-de-militantes-na-ditadura.html.

34. Juan Arias, "Los Médicos de Brasil 'Juzgan' a 26 Colegas por Colaborar con la Dictadura Militar" [Doctors in Brazil "judge" 26 colleagues for collaborating with the military dictatorship]," *El País*, March 4, 1999, https://elpais.com/diario/1999

/03/04/sociedad/920502003_850215.html; Lucas and Pross, "Caught between Conscience"; Nunca Máis, "Conselho Federal de Medicine cassa registro de medicos legistas" [Federation erases coroners from the registry], June 15, 2003.

35. "Julgamendo no conselho regional de medicina/SP" [Judgment at the Regional Council of Medicine/SP], *Jornal do Grupo Tortura Nunca Mais*, March 2000, 4, http://www.torturanuncamais-rj.org.br/jornal/gtnm_80/dia_internacional_lutra _contra_tortura.html.

36. "MPF quer responsabilizar agentes por tortura" [MPF wants to hold agents accountable for torture], *Consultor Jurídico*, March 3, 2009, https://www.conjur .com.br/2009-mar-03/mpf-responsabilizar-agentes-doi-tortura.

37. Cristina Grillo, "Conselho condena médico por participar de sessão de tortura" [Council condemns doctor for attending torture], *Folha de São Paulo*, March 5, 1999, https://www1.folha.uol.com.br/fsp/brasil/fc05039922.htm; Larry Rohter, "Brazil Rights Group Hopes to Bar Doctors Linked to Torture," *New York Times*, March 11, 1999, https://www.nytimes.com/1999/03/11/world /brazil-rights-group-hopes-to-bar-doctors-linked-to-torture.html; "Tribunal Regional Federal da 2 Região TRF-2- Apelação Civel: AC 200102010056828 RJ 2001.02.01.005682–8" [Federal Regional Court of the 2nd Region TRF-2- Civil Appeal: AC 200102010056828 RJ 2001.02.01.005682–8], February 1, 2001, *Jusbrasil*, https://trf-2.jusbrasil.com.br/jurisprudencia/6403486/apelacao-civel-ac -200102010056828-rj-20010201005682–8/inteiro-teor-12519734.

38. "Médico Acusado de Ligação com Tortura e Julgado" [Physician accused of torture is judged], *Folha De São Paulo*, August 10, 1995, http://www1.folha.uol.com .br/fsp/1995/8/10/brasil/30.html.

39. Robert S. Wallerstein, "The Intersect of Psychoanalysis and Totalitarianism," *Psychoanalytic Dialogues* 24 (October 17, 2014): 601–14, https://doi.org/10.1080 /10481885.2014.949495; Lucia Villela, "The Chalice of Silence and the Case That Refuses to Go Away," *Psychoanalytic Review* 92, no. 6 (December 2005): 807–28, https://doi.org/10.1521/prev.2005.92.6.807; Cristina Grillo, "Médico Amílcar Lobo Morre Aos 58 no Rio" [Doctor Amílcar Lobo dies at 58 in Rio], *Folha de São Paulo*, August 23, 1997, http://www1.folha.uol.com.br/fsp/brasil/fc230815.htm.

40. Amnesty International, *Brazil: "They Treat Us like Animals": Torture and Ill-Treatment in Brazil: Dehumanization and Impunity within the Criminal Justice System*, AMR 19/022/2001, October 17, 2001, https://www.amnesty.org/en/documents /amr19/022/2001/en/.

41. Wolfgang S. Heinz and Hugo Frühling, *Determinants of Gross Human Rights Violations by State and State Sponsored Actors in Brazil, Uruguay, Chile and Argentina: 1960–1990* (London: Martinus Nijhoff, 1999).

42. Colegio Médico de Chile, "The Participation of Physicians in Torture," in Stover, *Open Secret*; and Francisco S. Rivas, *Traición a Hipócrates: Médicos en el Apárato Represivo de la Dictadura* [Treason to Hippocrates: Doctors in the repressive apathy of the dictatorship] (Santiago: Ediciones Chile-América CESOC, 1990), http://www.blest.eu/biblio/rivas/index.html.

43. Juan San Cristóbal, "Los Médicos de la Dictadura que Ejercen en la Impunidad" [Doctors of the dictatorship have impunity], *Diario Uchile*, August 26,

2013, http://radio.uchile.cl/2013/08/26/los-medicos-de-la-dictadura-que-ejercen-en-la-impunidad/; Memoria Viva-Ethics Commission against Torture, "A Digital Archive of Those Who Violated Human Rights during the Military Dictatorship in Chile, 1973–1990," *Chile: Colonia del Neoliberalismo* (blog), September 25, 2011, https://radiochile-canada.net/2011/09/25/sale-a-la-luz-el-listado-de-los-medicos-que-torturaron-durante-la-dictadura-de-pinochet/. [Warning: very graphic image.]

44. Amnesty International, *Human Rights in Chile: The Role of the Medical Profession* (New York: Amnesty International, 1986); National Research Council Committee on Human Rights, *Scientists and Human Rights in Chile: Report of a Delegation* (Washington, DC: National Academies Press, 1985); Gunther Seelmann, "The Position of the Chilean Medical Association with Respect to Torture as an Instrument of Political Repression," *Journal of Medical Ethics*, S17 (December 1, 1991): 33–34, https://doi.org/10.1136/jme.17.Suppl.33; San Cristóbal, "Los médicos de la dictadura"; Centro de Estudios Miguel Enriquez, "Funado Camilo Azar Médico torturador" [Camilo Azar medical torturer], Archivo Chile, December 2003, http://www.archivochile.com/Derechos_humanos/FUNA/hhddfuna0038.pdf; Juan Luís González, "The Work of the Medical Association of Chile," in *Science and Human Rights*, ed. Carol Carillon (Washington, DC: National Academies Press, 1988), 1–106, https://www.nap.edu/catalog/9733/science-and-human-rights; and Rivas, *Traición a Hipócrates*.

45. Rivas; Brian Goldman, "Chilean Medical College Battles Doctor Participating in Torture," *Canadian Medical Association Journal* 132, no. 12 (June 15, 1985): 1414–16, http://www.ncbi.nlm.nih.gov/pmc/articles/PMC1346112/; and DCHpress, "Asesinato del Mayor de ejército, Carlos Hernán Pérez Castro y de su cónyuge, Anita Luisa Schlager Casanueva" [Assassination of army major Carlos Hernán Pérez Castro and his spouse Anita Luisa Schlager Casanueva], *Despierta Chile* (blog), March 3, 2008, https://despiertachile.wordpress.com/2008/03/03/ocurrio-un-3-de-marzo/.

46. Proyecto Internacional de Derechos Humanos [International Human Rights Project], "Manfred Jurgensen Caesar: Medicina General, Colaborador de la CNI" [Manfred Jurgensen Caesar: Internist, collaborator of CNI], Memoria Viva, accessed August 6, 2018, http://www.memoriaviva.com/criminales/criminales_j/jurgensen_manfred.htm; and Proyecto Internacional de Derechos Humanos, "Luis Alberto Losada Fuenzalida: Medico Cirujano, Colaborador de la CNI" [Luis Alberto Losada Fuenzalida: Surgeon, collaborator of CNI], Memoria Vivia, accessed August 6, 2018, http://www.memoriaviva.com/criminales/criminales_l/losada_luis.htm.

47. Proyecto Internacional de Derechos Humanos, "Camilo Azar Saba: Medico Traumatologo and Orthopedista, Torturador, Colaborador de la CNI" [Camilo Azar Saba: Traumatologist and orthopedic surgeon, torturer, collaborator of CNI], Memoria Vivia, accessed August 6, 2018, http://www.memoriaviva.com/criminales/criminales_a/azar_camilo.htm.

48. Proyecto Internacional de Derechos Humanos, "Víctor Domingo Carcuro Correa: Medico/Pediatra, Colaborador de la CNI" [Víctor Domingo Carcuro Correa: Pediatrician, collaborator of CNI]," Memoria Viva, accessed August 6,

2018, http://www.memoriaviva.com/criminales/criminales_c/carcuro_correa_victor.htm.

49. Proyecto Internacional de Derechos Humanos, "Guido Mario Felix Diaz Paci, Medico del Ejercito, Agente CNI" [Guido Mario Felix Diaz Paci, expelled doctor, agent of CNI], Memoria Viva, accessed August 6, 2018, http://www.memoriaviva.com/criminales/criminales_d/diaz_paci_guido.htm.

50. "Colegio Médico Expulsa del Gremio a Doctor Acusado de Torturas" [Colegio Médico expels a doctor accused of torture], *El Mercurio*, October 4, 2005, http://www.emol.com/noticias/nacional/2005/10/04/197311/colegio-medico-expulsa-del-gremio-a-doctor-acusado-de-torturas.html; and Santiago Appeals Court, July 20, 2010, www.observatorioluzibarburu.org/media/uploads/218298.pdf.

51. Proyecto Internacional de Derechos Humanos, "Torturers, Collaborators and Accomplices," Memoria Viva, accessed August 6, 2018, http://www.memoriaviva.com/English/criminals_list.htm; and "Solo, Abandonado Y Loco, Como Merecía, Murió el Hiptonizador and Torturador Osvaldo Pincetti" [Alone, abandoned and crazy, as he deserved, the hypnotist and torturer Osvaldo Pincetti died], *Zona Impacto*, June 12, 2007, http://www.zonaimpacto.cl/205/solo-abandonado-y-loco-como-merecia-murio-el-hiptonizador-y-torturador-osvaldo-pincetti.html.

52. Proyecto Internacional de Derechos Humanos, "José Maria Fuentealba Suazo, Medico del Ejercito" [José Maria Fuentealba Suazo, army doctor], Memoria Viva, accessed August 6, 2018, http://www.memoriaviva.com/criminales/criminales_f/fuentealba_jose.htm.

53. "Report 'Never Again': National Commission on the Disappearance of Persons (CONADEP)," Derecho Humanos, September 1984, http://www.derechoshumanos.net/lesahumanidad/informes/argentina/informe-de-la-CONADEP-Nunca-mas-Indice.htm#C6.

54. Luis Justo, "Argentina: Torture, Silence and Medical Teaching," *British Medical Journal* 326 (2003): 1405, https://iahponline.wordpress.com/2003/07/27/argentina-torture-silence-and-medical-teaching/.

55. Diana R. Kordon, "Impunity's Psychological Effects: Its Ethical Consequences," *Journal of Medical Ethics* S17 (December 1, 1991): 29–32, https://doi.org/10.1136/jme.17.Suppl.29.

56. Lucas and Pross, "Caught between Conscience"; Nunca Máis, "Conselho Federal de Medicine."

57. "Doctor, a Torturer, Is Shot in Argentina," *New York Times*, April 7, 1996, https://www.nytimes.com/1996/04/07/world/doctor-a-torturer-is-shot-in-argentina.html; and Adriana Meyer, "Condenas de Hasta 18 Anos a la ORP que Atacó a Bergés" [Sentences of up to 18 years to the ORP those who attacked Bergés], *Página 12*, April 25, 2002, https://www.pagina12.com.ar/diario/elpais/1-4415-2002-04-25.htm.

58. "Otorgan Domiciliaria con Tobillera al Genocida Jorge Héctor Vidal" [Home arrest for genocidal Jorge Héctor Vidal], *Red Eco Alternativo*, December 20, 2017, http://www.redeco.com.ar/nacional/ddhh/22923-otorgan-domiciliaria-con-tobillera-al-genocida-jorge-h%C3%A9ctor-vidal.

59. Ailín Bullentini, "La Pata Sanitaria del Terror Estatal" [The sanitary claw of state terror], *Página 12*, April 16, 2012, https://www.pagina12.com.ar/diario/elpais/1-191951-2012-04-16.html; Luis Justo, "Argentina: Torture, Silence, and Medical Teaching," *British Medical Journal* 326, no. 7403 (June 21, 2003): 1405, https://doi.org/10.1136/bmj.326.7403.1405; and Edward Schumacher, "Argentina Torture: One Who Looked On," *New York Times*, January 28, 1984, https://www.nytimes.com/1984/01/28/world/argentina-torture-one-who-looked-on.html.

60. "Rechazan la Acusación Contra Rodríguez Varela," *The Nation*, December 22, 2012, https://www.lanacion.com.ar/1539579-rechazan-la-acusacion-contra-rodriguez-varela.

61. Camile Cagni and Julio Ferrer, "Néstor Siri: Un Médico del Infierno" [Néstor Siri: A doctor from hell], *Voltaire Network*, May 8, 2006, http://www.voltairenet.org/article138564.html; and "Suspension para el Repressor" [Suspension for the torturer], *Página 12*, January 28, 2006, https://www.pagina12.com.ar/diario/elpais/1-62231-2006-01-28.html.

62. "Represores Argentinos: Agatino Federico Di Benedetto" [Argentine torturers: Agatino Federico di Benedetto], *Desaparecidos*, http://www.desaparecidos.org/arg/tort/ejercito/dibenedetto/; and "El Centro Clandestino Del Hospital," *Página 12*, October 20, 2011, https://www.pagina12.com.ar/diario/elpais/1-179278-2011-10-20.html.

63. "Argentina Jails 'Dirty War' Medic," BBC News, April 23, 2005, http://news.bbc.co.uk/2/hi/americas/4475693.stm; Alejandro Rebossio, "Los 11 Acusados por el Robo de Bebés en la Dictadura Argentina" [The 11 accused of the theft of babies during the Argentine dictatorship], *El País Internacional*, July 5, 2012, https://elpais.com/internacional/2012/07/05/actualidad/1341485352_811774.html; and "Confirman condena al médico naval Jorge Magnacco, que atendia partos en 'La Sardá' de la ESMA" [Conviction of the navy doctor Jorge Magnacco, who attended deliveries in 'la Sardá' of the ESMA], Télam: Agencia Nacional de Noticias, July 3, 2013, http://memoria.telam.com.ar/noticia/confirman-condena-a-un-medico-de-la-esma_n2750.

64. Uki Goñi, "Sins of the Father: Daughters of Men Who Killed for Argentina's Regime Speak Out," *Guardian*, June 13, 2017, https://www.theguardian.com/world/2017/jun/13/argentina-daughters-military-dictatorship-father.

65. "Bignone Reynaldo Procesamiento Prisi Preventiva" [Bignone case, Reynaldo B. and others processing and preventive prison], *V|Lex*, Exp. No. 16,964 / 08 Reg. No. 1165, October 27, 2009, https://ar.vlex.com/vid/bignone-reynaldo-procesamiento-prisi-preventiva-70379946.

66. "Murió el coronel retirado Arias Duval, que en Sociedad con Camps sembrómuerte y destrucción en La Plata" [Colonel Arias Duval died, who in partnership with camps sowed death and destruction in La Plata], Télam: Agencia Nacional de Noticias, May 28, 2012, http://memoria.telam.com.ar/noticia/murio-el-coronel-retirado-agustin—el-gato—arias-duval_n1112.

67. "Condenaron a los represores (neuquen)" [They condemned the repressors (Neuquén)], *Taringa!*, December 19, 2008, https://www.taringa.net/posts/noticias/1895953/Condenaron-a-los-represores-neuquen.html; "Condenaron con Penas de Entre 6 y 25 Años de Prisión a los Reprosores Jazgados en Neuquén"

[Condemned with sentences of between 6 and 25 years to prison the torturers repressors tried in Neuquén], Télam: Agencia Nacional de Noticias, May 14, 2014, http://www.telam.com.ar/notas/201405/63124-tribunal-oral-en-lo-criminal -federal-neuquen-juicio-oral-dictadura-civico-militar.html.

68. Ailín Bullentini, "Cuatro Condenas por Apropiación de Niños" [Four sentences for kidnapping children], *Página 12*, December 23, 2014, https://www.pagina12 .com.ar/diario/elpais/1-262537-2014-12-23.html; Jeremy H. Baron, "Genocidal Doctors," *Journal of the Royal Society of Medicine* 92, no. 11 (November 1, 1999): 590–93, https://doi.org/10.1177/014107689909201117; Alejandro Rebossio, "La ESMA Fue el Único Lugar Donde se Torturaba Por Placer" [ESMA was the only place where you tortured for pleasure], *El País Internacional*, November 30, 2012, https://elpais.com/internacional/2012/11/30/actualidad/1354297594_544752 .html; Cecilia Devanna, "Maternidad ilegal de Campo de Mayo: Condenan a Un Médico y Una Obstetra" [Illegal obstetrics ward at Campo de Mayo: A doctor and obstetrician are condemned], Infojus Noticias, December 22, 2014, http:// www.infojusnoticias.gov.ar/nacionales/maternidad-ilegal-de-campo-de-mayo -condenan-a-un-medico-y-una-obstetra-6900.html.

69. Cámara Federal de Mendoza, *Sentencia de Cámara Federal de Apelaciones de Mendoza*, FMZ 62000727/2012/5/CA1, December 22, 2014, https://ar.vlex.com/vid /legajo-n-5-imputado-557757714.

70. "Las Abuelos Recuperaron a la 90 Nieta," El Pais, Télam, May 29, 2008, http:// diarioepoca.com/170515/Abuelas-recuperaron-a-la-nieta-numero-90/.

71. Carlos R. Capella, "9 Perpetuas and 1 Absuelto de 29 Procesados" [9 life sentences and one acquitted of 29 processed], *La Noticia*, April 13, 2015, http:// lanoticiasl.com/noticia.php?id=1288.

72. Marias Gatcias Elorria, "Lesa humanidad: 28 condenados y un absuelto en el juicio por-crimenes en San Luis" [Laws of humanity: 28 convicted and one acquitted in the trial in San Luis], *El Diario de La Republica* (Argentina), April 10, 2015, https://www.eldiariodelarepublica.com/nota/2015-4-10-14-26 -0-lesa-humanidad-28-condenados-y-un-absuelto-en-el-juicio-por-crimenes -en-san-luis.

73. Gary Marx, "For Children of 'Disappeared,' a Different Torture," *Chicago Tribune*, April 4, 1993, http://articles.chicagotribune.com/1993-04-04/news /9304040227_1_biological-families-identity-twins-parents; and Barbara Crossette, "DNA Test Reunites Salvadoran Mother and Child," *New York Times*, January 21, 1995, https://www.nytimes.com/1995/01/21/world/dna-test-reunites -salvadoran-mother-and-child.html.

74. "Condenan a militar retirado por apropiación de un bebé" [A retired military man condemned for kidnapping a baby], *El Ciudadano*, September 9, 2014, https:// www.elciudadanoweb.com/condenan-a-militar-retirado-por-apropiacion-de-un -bebe/.

75. Devanna, "No sé para que."

76. Associated Press, "Argentine Church Will Hand over Certificates for Baptisms Performed at Torture Chamber," *Catholic Herald*, March 7, 2018, http:// www.catholicherald.co.uk/news/2018/03/07/argentine-church-will-hand-over -certificates-for-baptisms-performed-at-torture-chamber/.

77. "Listado de Medicos Relacionados con la Represion; del period 1976 a 1983 en Argentina" [List of doctors related to repression: From the period 1976 to 1983 in Argentina], Grupo Fahrenheit [Fahrenheit Group], accessed August 6, 2018, http://www.desaparecidos.org/GrupoF/medicos.html.

78. Daniel Riera, "Algo de Justicia: Condenan a Tres Policías que Abusaron de un Joven en Trelew" [Some justice: Three policemen who abused a young man in Trelew are condemned], *Big Bang News*, April 23, 2016, https://www.bigbangnews.com/policiales/Algo-de-Justicia-condenan-a-tres-policias-que-abusaron-de-un-joven-en-Trelew-20160423–0015.html.

79. "Si no hay justicia, hay escrache!" [If there is no justice, there is demonstration!], *Indymedia*, December 2, 2003, http://archivo.argentina.indymedia.org/news/2003/12/155329.php; Martín Cúneo, "Si no hay justicia, hay escrache" [If there is no justice, there is denouncing], *Diagonal*, February 13, 2013, https://www.diagonalperiodico.net/global/si-no-hay-justicia-hay-escrache.html; and Karina Rojas, "Si no hay justicia, hay escrache!," *Laizquierda Diario*, December 17, 2014, https://www.laizquierdadiario.com.uy/Montevideo-Si-no-hay-justicia-hay-escrache.

## Chapter 12: Globalization

1. Steven H. Miles, Telma Alencar, and Britney Crock, "Punishing Physicians Who Torture: A Work in Progress," *Torture* 20, no. 1 (2010): 23–31, https://irct.org/assets/uploads/Punishing+physicians.pdf.

2. Michael Schwirtz, "In Russia, Charges Are Dropped in Jail Death," *New York Times*, April 8, 2012, https://www.nytimes.com/2012/04/09/world/europe/russia-drops-charges-against-doctor-in-jail-death.html.

3. Miriam Elder, "Russian Court Clears Doctor over Sergei Magnitsky's Death in Custody," *Guardian*, December 28, 2012, http://www.theguardian.com/world/2012/dec/28/russian-doctor-sergei-magnitsky-death; Schwirtz, "In Russia, Charges Are Dropped."

4. "Premio a Toccafondi, medico 'torturatore' del G8: la replica della Asl 3 Genovese" [Award to Toccafondi, doctor 'torturer' of the G8: The reply of the Asl 3 Genovese], Genova24.it, July 15, 2011, http://www.genova24.it/2011/07/premio-a-toccafondi-medico-%E2%80%9Ctorturatore%E2%80%9D-del-g8-la-replica-della-asl-3-genovese-16521/; European Union, *Charter of Fundamental Rights of the European Union*, 2012/C 326/02, https://eur-lex.europa.eu/legal-content/EN/TXT/?uri=CELEX:12012P/TXT.

5. Marco Preve, "G8: professione disonorata, quei medici vanno radiati" [G8: Dishonored profession, those doctors must be removed], *La Repubblica*, August 7, 2013, http://genova.repubblica.it/cronaca/2013/08/07/news/g8_professione_disonorata_quei_medici_vanno_radiati-64400895/.

6. "'Stefano Cucchi è morto per malnutrizone': Ecco le motivazioni della condanna dei medici" ["Stefano Cucchi died of malnutrition": Here are the reasons for the condemnation of the doctors], *La Repubblica Romana.it*, September 3, 2013, https://roma.repubblica.it/cronaca/2013/09/03/news/stefano_cucchi_morto_per

_malnutrizione_depositate_motivazioni_della_condanna_dei_medici-65802108/;
Carlo Picozza, "'Stefano non è stato alimentato né idratato': Il mistero degli ultimi
suoi giorni al 'Pertini'" ["Stefano was not fed or hydrated": The mystery of his
last days at "Pertini"], *La Repubblica*, November 2, 2009, http://www.repubblica
.it/2009/10/sezioni/cronaca/morte-cucchi/cucchi-non-anoressico/cucchi-non
-anoressico.html; and Silvia di Carlo, "Stefano Cucchi, motivazioni assoluzione
medici: 'Morte per inanizione. Non si sarebbe salvato.' Ilaria: 'Indignata'" [Stefano
Cucchi, medical absolution motivations: "Death by inanition. He would not save
himself." Ilaria: "Outraged"], *Il Fatto Quotidiano*, October 7, 2016, https://www
.ilfattoquotidiano.it/2016/10/07/stefano-cucchi-motivazioni-assoluzione-medici
-morte-per-inanizione-non-si-sarebbe-salvato/3081634/.

7. "Iraqi Doctor Suspended over Torture Links," BBC News, March 1, 2013,
https://www.bbc.com/news/uk-21633391.

8. Jagdish C. Sobti, B. C. Chapparaawal, and Erik Holst, "Study of Knowledge, Attitude, and Practices concerning Aspects of Torture," *Journal of the Indian Medical
Association* 98, no. 6 (2000): 334–35, 338–39.

9. "Controversy Erupts Again over Kalinga Nagar Victims," *Outlook India*, January 13, 2006, https://www.outlookindia.com/newswire/story/controversy-erupts
-again-over-kalinga-nagar-victims/348354.

10. "Sri Lanka: Medical Council Erases the Name of a Doctor for Three Years for
Failure to Properly Carry Out His Duties in Examining a Torture Victim," Asian
Human Rights Commission, August 6, 2007, http://www.humanrights.asia/news
/ahrc-news/AS-181–2007.

11. "Sri Lanka: Officers."

12. "Jail Doctor Charged with Inmate's Torture," *Daily Times*, October 18, 2008.

13. Amnesty International, *Health Crisis Syrian Government Targets the Wounded and
Health Workers*, MDE 24/059/2011, October 25, 2011, https://www.amnesty.org
/en/documents/mde24/059/2011/en/.

14. "Doctor Fined over Inaccurate Report on Tortured Woman in Turkey's West,"
*Hürriyet Daily News* (Istanbul), July 6, 2015, http://www.hurriyetdailynews.com
/doctor-fined-over-inaccurate-report-on-tortured-woman-in-turkeys-west-85036.

15. El Shafi Beshir, "How to Struggle against Torture," *Journal of Medical Ethics*
S17, no. 1 (December 1991): 62–63, https://www.ncbi.nlm.nih.gov/pmc/articles
/PMC1378180/.

16. Abdel-Rahman Hussein, "Egyptian Army Doctor Cleared over 'Virginity Tests'
on Women Activists," *Guardian*, March 11, 2012, https://www.theguardian.com
/world/2012/mar/11/egypt-doctor-cleared-virginity-tests.

17. Fady Salah, "Tahrir Doctors File Complaint against FJP Member," *Daily News*,
December 12, 2012, https://dailynewsegypt.com/2012/12/12/tahrir-doctors-file
-complaint-against-fjp-member/; Aswat Masriya, "Muslim Brotherhood Figures
Sentenced to 15 Years for Torture," *Egyptian Streets*, October 11, 2014, https://
egyptianstreets.com/2014/10/11/muslim-brotherhood-figures-sentenced-to-15
-years-for-torture/.

18. Sikkink, *Justice Cascade*, 96–129; Méndez and Wentworth, *Taking a Stand*, 137–
85; Hayner, *Unspeakable Truths*.

19. "Mau Mau Torture Victims to Receive Compensation—Hague," BBC News, June 6, 2013, https://www.bbc.com/news/uk-22790037.
20. George Annas, "Medical Ethics and Human Rights in Wartime," *South African Medical Journal* 105, no. 4 (April 2015): 240, https://https://doi.org/10.7196/SAMJ.9529.
21. World Health Organization, *Health Workforce Requirements for Universal Health Coverage and the Sustainable Development Goals*, 2016, 3–23, http://apps.who.int/iris/bitstream/handle/10665/250330/9789241511407-eng.pdf.
22. "Physicians (per 1000 People)," World Bank, accessed January 15, 2019, https://data.worldbank.org/indicator/sh.med.phys.zs.
23. Mia Malan, "Dr. Death Close to Patients' Hearts," Bhekisisa: Centre for Health Journalism, November 22, 2013, http://mg.co.za/article/2013-11-22-dr-death-close-to-patients-hearts.

## Chapter 13. Impunity and the US War on Terror

1. Institute on Medicine as a Profession, *Ethics Abandoned: Medical Professionalism and Detainee Abuse in the "War on Terror"* (Washington, DC: Institute on Medicine as a Profession, 2013), http://imapny.org/wp-content/themes/imapny/File%20Library/Documents/IMAP-EthicsTextFinal2.pdf; Constitution Project Task Force, *The Report of the Constitution Projects Task Force on Detainee Treatment* (Washington, DC: Constitution Project, 2013), https://detaineetaskforce.org/report/download/; Farnoosh Hashemian, *Broken Law, Broken Lives: Medical Evidence of Torture by U.S. Personnel and Its Impact* (New York: PHR, 2008), http://physiciansforhumanrights.org/library/reports/broken-laws-torture-report-2008.html; Scott A. Allen, *Leave No Marks: Enhanced Interrogation Techniques and the Risk of Criminality* (New York: PHR, 2007), http://physiciansforhumanrights.org/library/reports/leave-no-marks-report-2007.html; Vincent Iacopino and Stephen N. Xenakis, "Neglect of Medical Evidence of Torture in Guantánamo Bay: A Case Series," *PLOS Medicine* 8, no. 4 (April 26, 2011), https://doi.org/10.1371/journal.pmed.1001027; Miles, *Oath Betrayed*; PHR, *Aiding Torture: Health Professionals' Ethics and Human Rights Violations Revealed in the May 2004 CIA Inspector General's Report*, 2009, http://physiciansforhumanrights.org/library/reports/aiding-torture-2009.html; PHR, *Experiments in Torture: Evidence of Human Subject Research and Experimentation in the "Enhanced" Interrogation Program*, 2010, http://physiciansforhumanrights.org/library/reports/experiments-in-torture-2010.html; Maxwell G. Bloche, *The Hippocratic Myth* (New York: Palgrave Macmillan, 2011), 119–57; Robert J. Lifton, "Doctors and Torture," *New England Journal of Medicine* 351, no. 5 (July 2004): 415–16, https://doi.org/10.1056/NEJMp048065; Steven H. Miles, "Abu Ghraib: Its Legacy for Military Medicine," *Lancet* 364, no. 9435 (August 21, 2004): 4725–29, https://doi.org/10.1016/S0140–6736(04)16902-X; Miles and Marks, "United States Military Medicine."
2. David Cole, *The Torture Memos: Rationalizing the Unthinkable* (New York: New Press, 2009).

3. "Humane Treatment of Al Qaeda and Taliban Detainees," White House Office of the Press Secretary, February 7, 2002, https://www.aclu.org/legal -document/presidential-memo-feb-7–2002-humane-treatment-al-qaeda-and -taliban-detainees.

4. "Statement of President Barack Obama on Release of OLC Memos," White House Office of the Press Secretary, April 16, 2009, https://obamawhitehouse .archives.gov/realitycheck/the-press-office/statement-president-barack-obama -release-olc-memos (emphasis added).

5. ICRC, *Third Geneva Convention*.

6. Emma Roller and Rebecca Nelson, "What CIA Interrogators Did to 17 Detainees without Approval," *Atlantic*, December 10, 2014, https://www.theatlantic.com /politics/archive/2014/12/what-cia-interrogators-did-to-17-detainees-without -approval/451281/.

7. Steven H. Miles, "Medical Investigations of Homicides of Prisoners of War in Iraq and Afghanistan," *Medscape* 7, no. 3 (2005): https://www.ncbi.nlm.nih.gov/pmc /articles/PMC1681676/; Miles, *Oath Betrayed*, 68–96.

8. US Department of Defense, *Working Group Report*, 52–56, 68–69.

9. Steven G. Bradbury, memorandum for John A. Rizzo, CIA, July 20, 2007, 6, https://www.justice.gov/olc/file/886296/download; CIA, *Summary and Reflections of Chief of Medical Services on OMS Participation in the RDI [Rendition, Detention, and Interrogation] Program*, 2007, https://www.aclu.org/report/summary-and -reflections-chief-medical-services-oms-participation-rdi-program.

10. Select Committee on Intelligence, Committee Study of the Central Intelligence Agency's Detention and Interrogation Program, S. Rep. No. 113–288, at 11 (2014), https://www.documentcloud.org/documents/1376748-sscistudy1.html.

11. Steven G. Bradbury, memorandum for John A. Rizzo, CIA, May 10, 2005, 14, https://fas.org/irp/agency/doj/olc/techniques.pdf.

12. CIA, *Summary and Reflections*, 39.

13. CIA, 41.

14. Paul Kramer, "The Water Cure: Debating Torture and Counterinsurgency— A Century Ago," *New Yorker*, February 25, 2008, https://www.newyorker.com /magazine/2008/02/25/the-water-cure.

15. Miles, *Oath Betrayed*, 148–51.

16. CIA, *Summary and Reflections*, 28.

17. Neil A. Lewis, "Red Cross Finds Detainee Abuse in Guantánamo," *New York Times*, November 30, 2004; "Re: GTMO," email, July 31, 2004, http://www.aclu .org/torturefoia/released/t3186_3187.pdf; Gretchen Borchelt, *Break Them Down: Systematic Use of Psychological Torture by U.S. Forces* (New York: PHR, 2005), 47, http://physiciansforhumanrights.org/library/reports/us-torture-break-them-down -2005.html.

18. UN Commission Economic and Security Council, *Situation of Detainees at Guantánamo Bay*, E/CN.4/2006/120 (February 27, 2006), 22, https://www.refworld .org/docid/45377b0b0.html; Borchelt, *Break Them Down*; Scott Shane and Mark Mazzetti, "In Adopting Harsh Tactics, No Inquiry into Their Past Use," *New York Times*, April 22, 2009, http://www.nytimes.com/2009/04/22/us/politics/22detain

.html; and James Risen and Matt Apuzzo, "CIA, on Path to Torture, Chose Haste over Analysis," *New York Times*, December 15, 2004, http://www.nytimes.com /2014/12/16/us/politics/cia-on-path-to-torture-chose-haste-over-analysis-.html.

19. Miles, *Oath Betrayed*, 186–99; James Risen, *Pay Any Price: Greed, Power, and Endless War* (New York: Houghton Mifflin Harcourt, 2014), 193–200.

20. *Report of the American Psychological Association Presidential Task Force on Psychological Ethics and National Security* (Washington, DC: American Psychological Association, June 2005); Steven H. Miles, *Oath Betrayed*, 186–99.

21. OTSG/MEDCOM, "Behavioral Science Consultation Policy," Policy Memo 06–029, October 20, 2006, http://humanrights.ucdavis.edu/projects/the -guantanamo-testimonials-project/testimonies/testimonies-of-standard-operating -procedures/behavioral_science_consultation_policy_memo_2006.pdf.

22. Sheri Fink, "Where Even Nightmares Are Classified: Psychiatric Care at Guantánamo," *New York Times*, November 12, 2016, https://www.nytimes.com/2016 /11/13/world/guantanamo-bay-doctors-abuse.html; and Iacopino and Xenakis, "Neglect of Medical Evidence."

23. Neil A. Lewis, "Guantanamo Tour Focuses on Medical Ethics," *New York Times*, November 13, 2005, http://www.nytimes.com/2005/11/13/national/13gitmo.html.

24. Secret Orcon [Origin Confidential], "Interrogation Log, Detainee 063," https:// content.time.com/time/2006/log/log.pdf; US Army, "First Special Interrogation Plan," in *Final Report: Investigation into FBI Allegations of Detainee Abuse at Guantanamo Bay, Cuba Detention Facility*, June 5, 2005, 13–21; CTD Fly Team, "Interviews," American Civil Liberties Union, various dates, http://www.aclu.org /torturefoia/legaldocuments/july_docs/(M)%20schmidt-furlow%20deferred .pdf; *GTMO Investigation—FBI Allegations of Abuse* [interviews of various dates], AR 15–6 Report, July 14, 2005, http://www1.umn.edu/humanrts/OathBetrayed /Schmidt-Furlow%20Report%20Enclosures%20II.pdf; Miles, *Oath Betrayed*, xvi– xviii, 169–85; Steven H. Miles, "Medical Ethics and the Interrogation of Guantanamo 063," *American Journal of Bioethics* 7, no. 4 (May 2007): 1–7; M. Gregg Bloche and Jonathan H. Marks, "Doctors and Interrogators at Guantanamo Bay," *New England Journal of Medicine* 353, no. 1 (July 2005): 6–8, https://doi.org/10 .1056/NEJMp058145.

25. Bradley Olson and Steven H. Miles, "The American Psychological Association and War on Terror Interrogations," in Miles, *Oath Betrayed*, 186–98; Psychologists for Social Responsibility, http://www.psysr.org/.

26. American Psychological Association, *Report of the Independent Reviewer and Related Materials*, last revised September 4, 2015, http://www.apa.org/independent-review/.

27. Andrea Korte, "2015 AAAS Scientific Freedom and Responsibility Award Goes to Social Psychologist Jean Maria Arrigo," *American Association of Science News*, February 8, 2016, https://www.aaas.org/news/2015-aaas-scientific-freedom-and -responsibility-award-goes-social-psychologist-jean-maria.

28. "Hoffman and Sidley Austin's Key Conclusions are Demonstrably False," http:// www.hoffmanreportapa.com/.

29. Sheri Fink, "Settlement Reached in C.I.A. Torture Case," *New York Times*, August 17, 2017, https://www.nytimes.com/2017/08/17/us/cia-torture-lawsuit -settlement.html.

30. Al Nasheri v. Romania, No. 33234/12, Eur Ct HR (2018); Abu Zubaydah v. Lith-uania, No. 46454/11, Eur Ct HR (2018); Al Nasheri v. Poland, No. 28761/11, Eur Ct HR (2014); Husayn (Abu Zubaydah) v. Poland, No. 7511/13 Eur Ct HR (2014).

31. Jim L. H. Cox, Dicky Grigg, and Joseph Margulies, "Complaint against James Elmer Mitchell," Texas State Board of Examiners of Psychologists, June 16, 2010, http://hrp.law.harvard.edu/wp-content/uploads/2013/07/MIT-FINL.pdf; Andrew Welsh-Huggins, "Letter Turns Up Heat on Psychologist," *Washington Post*, July 11, 2010, http://www.washingtonpost.com/wp-dyn/content/article/2010/07/10/AR2010071002896.html; "Texas Board Won't Discipline CIA Psychologist," FoxNews Houston, February 25, 2011, http://www.myfoxhouston.com/story/18177122/texas-board-wont-discipline-cia-psychologist; Michael Reese, Trudy Bond, Colin Bossen, and Josephine Setzler, "Complaint form—Larry C. James, License No. 6492," State Board of Psychology of Ohio, July 7, 2010, http://hrp.law.harvard.edu/wp-content/uploads/2013/06/larry_james_6492.pdf; State Board of Psychology of Ohio, January 26, 2011, http://hrp.law.harvard.edu/wp-content/uploads/2013/06/james-letter31.pdf; Kathy Roberts, Nushin Sarkarati, and Andrea Evans, "Complaint—John Francis Leso, NY License # 013492," n.d., http://www.cja.org/article.php?id=876; Jonathon H. Marks, "The Silence of the Doctors," *TruthOut*, December 13, 2005, http://truth-out.org/archive/component/k2/item/59289:jonathan-h-marks—the-silence-of-the-doctors; Janice H. Tanne, "Lawyers Will Appeal Ruling That Cleared Guantanamo Doctor of Ethics Violations," *British Medical Journal* 331, no. 7510 (July 2005): 180, https://www.ncbi.nlm.nih.gov/pmc/articles/PMC1179805/; Center for Constitutional Rights, "The Case of Dr. Larry C. James," accessed June 10, 2019, https://ccrjustice.org/sites/default/files/assets/files/09.08.06_bond%20backgrounder%20FINAL.pdf; Dr. Trudy Bond v. Louisiana State Board of Examiners of Psychologists, State of Louisiana, Court of Appeals, First Circuit, CA1735, June 11, 2010, Justia US Law, https://law.justia.com/cases/louisiana/first-circuit-court-of-appeal/2010/2009ca1735-1.html; Deborah Popowski, "Beyond the APA: The Role of Psychology Boards and State Courts in Propping Up Torture," Justia Security, August 24, 2015, https://www.justsecurity.org/25378/apa-role-psychology-boards-state-courts-propping-torture/; and Roy J. Eidelson, "'No Cause for Action': Revisiting the Ethics Case of Dr. John Leso," *Journal of Social and Political Psychology* 3, no. 1 (2015): 198–212, https://doi.org/10.5964/jspp.v3i1.479.

32. Carol D. Goodheart, "Letter to Texas State Board of Psychologists," American Psychological Association, June 30, 2010, http://www.apa.org/news/press/statements/texas-mitchell-letter.pdf.

33. Leonard Rubenstein et al., "Coercive U.S. Interrogation Policies: A Challenge to Medical Ethics," *JAMA* 294, no. 12 (September 2005): 1544–49; Lawrence S. Rubenstein and Stephen N. Xenakis, "Roles of CIA Physicians in Enhanced Interrogation and Torture of Detainees," *JAMA* 304, no. 12 (August 2010): 569–70.

34. Susan Mayor, "Medical Bodies Urge Investigation of Alleged Involvement in Torture," *British Medical Journal* 329, no. 7464 (2004): 473, https://www.ncbi.nlm.nih.gov/pmc/articles/PMC515222/.

35. P. Peck, "AMA Asks Bush for Iraq Prison Inquiry," UPI, June 14, 2004.

36. ICRC, *Report on the Treatment by the Coalition Forces of Prisoners of War and Other Protected Persons by the Geneva Conventions in Iraq during Arrest, Internment and Interrogation*, February 2004, http://cryptome.org/icrc-report.htm; UN Human Rights Council, Observations on Communications Transmitted to Governments and Replies Received, A/HRC/31/57/Add.1 (February 24, 2016), 105–6, https://www.ohchr.org/en/hrbodies/hrc/regularsessions/session31/pages/listreports.aspx; ICRC, *Report on the Treatment of Fourteen "High-Value Detainees" in CIA Custody*, 2007, https://www.globalsecurity.org/intell/library/reports/2007/icrc-report_hvd-cia-custody-2007.htm.

37. UN Commission on Human Rights, "Situation of Detainees at Guantánamo Bay," E/CN.4/2006/120 (February 27, 2006), http://repository.un.org/bitstream/handle/11176/259174/E_CN.4_2006_120-EN.pdf.

38. Andis Robeznieks, "Military Doctors Reminded of Wartime Roles," AMEDNEWS.com, September 27, 2004, https://amednews.com/article/20040927/profession/309279959/7/.

39. Robeznieks.

40. Select Committee on Intelligence, Committee Study.

41. Elise Viebeck, "AMA Rebukes Doctors for Role in CIA 'Torture,'" *The Hill*, December 12, 2014, http://thehill.com/policy/healthcare/227005-ama-rebukes-doctors-for-role-in-cia-torture.

42. PHR, *Doing Harm: Health Professionals' Central Role in the CIA Torture Program: Medical and Psychological Analysis of the 2014 U.S. Senate Select Committee on Intelligence Report's Executive Summary*, 2014, http://physiciansforhumanrights.org/library/reports/doing-harm-health-professionals-central-role-in-the-cia-torture-program.html.

43. Editorial Board, "Tortured by Psychologists and Doctors," *New York Times*, December 16, 2004, http://www.nytimes.com/2014/12/17/opinion/tortured-by-psychologists-and-doctors.html.

44. Brenden Moore, "DePaul Dean Gerald Koocher Implicated in Torture Report," *DePaulia*, August 21, 2015, https://depauliaonline.com/13843/news/depaul-dean-gerald-koocher-apa-torture/.

45. Tom Bartlett, "Psychologist Implicated in APA's Torture Report Resigns Academic Post," *Chronicle of Higher Education*, July 21, 2015, https://www.chronicle.com/blogs/ticker/psychologist-implicated-in-apas-torture-report-resigns-academic-post/102233.

46. "Psychologist Who Helped Devise CIA Interrogation Program Lost Mormon Role," Reuters, December 11, 2014, http://www.reuters.com/article/2014/12/12/us-usa-cia-torture-psychologists-idUSKBN0JQ00H20141212.

47. Colleen Flaherty, "Northern Arizona Won't Interview Former Army Psychologist with Ties to Abu Ghraib," *Inside Higher Education*, January 29, 2014, https://www.insidehighered.com/quicktakes/2014/01/29/northern-arizona-wont-interview-former-army-psychologist-ties-abu-ghraib.

48. WMA, *Resolution on the Responsibility of Physicians*.

49. "If the US Tortures, Why Can't We Do It?," UN Office of the High Commissioner of Human Rights, December 11, 2014, http://www.ohchr.org/EN/NewsEvents /Pages/DisplayNews.aspx?NewsID=15406&LangID=E.

## Chapter 14. Promoting Accountability

1. Amnesty International, *Torture in 2014: 30 Years of Broken Promises*, ACT 40/004/2014, 2014, https://www.amnestyusa.org/reports/torture-in-2014–30 -years-of-broken-promises/.

2. Amnesty International, *Attitudes to Torture*, ACT 40/005/2014, 2014, https://www .amnesty.org/en/documents/ACT40/005/2014/en/.

3. Jose Quiroga and James M. Jaranson, "Politically-Motivated Torture and Its Survivors," *Torture* 15, nos. 2–3 (January 2005): 1–112; Sondra S. Crosby et al., "Prevalence of Torture Survivors among Foreign-Born Patients Presenting to an Urban Ambulatory Care Practice," *Journal of General Internal Medicine* 21 (2006): 764–68; David Eisenman, Allen Keller, and G. Kim, "Survivors of Torture in a General Medical Setting: How Often Have Patients Been Tortured and How Often Is It Missed?," *Journal of Western Medicine* 172, no. 5 (May 2000): 301–4; Edith Montgomery and Anders Foldspang, "Criterion-Related Validity of Screening for Exposure to Torture," *Danish Medical Bulletin* 41, no. 5 (November 1994): 588–91; Masmas et al., "Asylum Seekers in Denmark," 77–86.

4. US Department of Justice, *Survivors of Politically Motivated Torture: A Large, Growing, and Invisible Population of Crime Victims*, January 2000, 1–14, https:// www.ncjrs.gov/App/Publications/abstract.aspx?ID=178911; Center for Victims of Torture, "U.S. Home to Far More Refugee Torture Survivors than Previously Believed," press release, September 29, 2015, https://www.cvt.org/news -events/press-releases/us-home-far-more-refugee-torture-survivors-previously -believed.

5. Daniel P. Mannix, *The History of Torture* (Stroud, UK: History Press, 1964); Lynn Hunt, *Inventing Human Rights* (New York: W. W. Norton, 2007), 76.

6. Petersen H. Draminsky, "Factor Interaction in Prevention of Torture: Reflections Based on Carver's and Handley's Research," *Torture* 27 (2007): 101–24, https:// www.ncbi.nlm.nih.gov/pubmed/30047494.

7. Sikkink, *Justice Cascade*; Méndez and Wentworth, *Taking a Stand*; Moyn, *Last Utopia*; Stephen Hopgood, *The Endtimes of Human Rights* (Ithaca, NY: Cornell University Press, 2013).

8. Jonathon M. Mann et al., eds., *Health and Human Rights: A Reader* (New York: Routledge, 1999), 11–18; Paul Farmer, *Pathologies of Power: Health, Human Rights, and the New War on the Poor* (Berkeley: University of California Press, 2005); Max Rosner, "Democracy," Our World in Data, 2019, https://ourworldindata .org/democracy; Center for the Advancement of Public Integrity, *The Corruption and Human Rights Connection* (New York: Columbia Law School, October 2018), https://www.law.columbia.edu/sites/default/files/microsites/public-integrity /the_corruption_and_human_rights_connection_4.pdf.

9. World Health Organization, *Violence and Injury Prevention*, 2018, http://www.who
   .int/violence_injury_prevention/violence/en/; World Health Organization, *Draft
   Global Plan of Action on Violence*, A69/9, March 11, 2016, http://apps.who.int/gb
   /ebwha/pdf_files/WHA69/A69_9-en.pdf.

10. World Health Association, "Appendix 2. Options for the Implementation of the
    Comprehensive Mental Health Action Plan, 2013–2020," in *Comprehensive Men-
    tal Health Action Plan: 2013–2020*, 2013, 21, http://apps.who.int/gb/ebwha/pdf
    _files/WHA66/A66_R8-en.pdf.

11. Danish Medical Association, "Doctors, Ethics and Torture," *Danish Medical Bul-
    letin* 34 (1987): 185–216; National Academy of Sciences, *Scientists and Human
    Rights in Chile: Report of a Delegation* (Washington, DC: National Academy of
    Sciences, 1985), http://books.nap.edu/openbook.php?record_id=9732&page=1.

12. David P. Forsythe, *Human Rights in International Relations* (Oxford: Cambridge
    University Press, 2012).

13. Oona Hathaway, "Do Human Rights Treaties Make a Difference?," *Yale Law
    Journal* 111 (January 2002): 1935–2042, http://digitalcommons.law.yale.edu/cgi
    /viewcontent.cgi?article=1852&context=fss_papers.

14. Mairi Mackay, "Torture Was Once 'Normal' in Georgia's Prisons—This Is
    How They 'Effectively Abolished' It," *Open Democracy*, July 28, 2016, https://
    www.opendemocracy.net/mairi-mackay/westminster/torture-georgia; "Georgia
    Has Come a Long Way, but More Needs to Be Done," UN Office of the High
    Commissioner for Human Rights, March 19, 2015, https://www.ohchr.org/EN
    /NewsEvents/Pages/DisplayNews.aspx?NewsID=15724.

15. Steven H. Miles, "Medical Associations and Accountability for Physician Par-
    ticipation in Torture," *American Medical Association Journal of Ethics* 17, no. 10
    (2015): 945–51, https://doi.org/10.1001/journalofethics.2015.17.10.pfor1–1510.

16. Magali Sarfatti Larson, *The Rise of Professionalism: A Sociological Analysis* (Berke-
    ley: University of California Press, 1978), 208.

17. Institute on Medicine as a Profession, *Ethics Abandoned*, 135–54.

18. UN Office of the High Commissioner of Human Rights, *Report on Encryp-
    tion, Anonymity, and the Human Rights Framework*, 2015, https://www.ohchr.org
    /en/issues/freedomopinion/pages/callforsubmission.aspx; "Promote Strong
    Encryption and Anonymity in the Digital Age," Human Rights Watch, June 17,
    2015, https://www.hrw.org/news/2015/06/17/promote-strong-encryption-and
    -anonymity-digital-age-0.

## Appendix: Behavioral Examples of Torture Doctoring

1. Canofre, "5 Accounts."

2. Reis et al., "Physician Participation," 1480–86.

3. ARCT, *Alternative Report*, 40.

4. "Analytical Study about the Leaked Pictures"; and UN Human Rights Council,
   Assault on Medical Care in Syria, A/HRC/24/CRP.2 (September 13, 2013), http://
   www.ohchr.org/EN/HRBodies/HRC/RegularSessions/Session24/_layouts/15

/WopiFrame.aspx?sourcedoc=/EN/HRBodies/HRC/RegularSessions/Session24
/Documents/A-HRC-24-CRP-2.doc.

5. Amnesty International, *Prisons within Prisons: Torture and Ill-Treatment of Prisoners of Conscience in Vietnam*, ASA 41/4187/2016, July 2016, 42, https://www
.amnestyusa.org/wp-content/uploads/2017/04/asa_4141872016_eng_report.pdf.

6. FIDH, *Mauritania: The Case of the 'Islamists': Torture in the Name of the Fight
against Terrorism*, September 2007, 20, https://www.fidh.org/IMG/pdf/Mauritanie
479ang.pdf.

7. Select Committee on Intelligence, Committee Study.

8. UN Economic and Social Council, Civil and Political Rights, Including: The
Questions of Torture and Detention: Mission to Mongolia, E/CN.4/2006/6/Add.4
(December 20, 2005), 21, https://documents-dds-ny.un.org/doc/UNDOC/GEN
/G05/167/32/PDF/G0516732.pdf.

9. Appellants v. State of Karnataka, Supreme Court of India, Criminal Appellate
Jurisdiction, No. 1267 of 2004.

10. Rejali, *Torture and Democracy*, 16–21.

11. Steven G. Bradbury, "Re: Application of United States Obligations under Article
16 of the Convention against Torture to Certain Techniques That May Be Used
in the Interrogation of High Value al Qaeda Detainees," memorandum for John A.
Rizzo, May 30, 2005, https://www.hsdl.org/?abstract&did=37511.

12. "Amputations in Sudan," *Amnesty International Newsletter* 14, no. 2 (February
1984): 1, https://www.amnesty.org/download/Documents/nws210021984en.pdf;
African Center for Justice and Peace Studies, "Sudan: Doctors Perform Amputations for Courts," February 27, 2013, http://www.acjps.org/?p=1317.

13. Amnesty International, *Amnesty International Report 2016/17*.

14. Kingsley and Loveluck, "Egyptian Doctors."

15. Dana Priest and Barton Gellman, "U.S. Decries Abuse but Defends Interrogations," *Washington Post*, December 26, 2002, http://www.washingtonpost.com/wp
-dyn/content/article/2006/06/09/AR2006060901356.html.

16. Jessica Dorfman, "Forced Sterilization in Uzbekistan," *Harvard International
Review*, January 21, 2014, http://hir.harvard.edu/article/?a=3206.

17. Abu Wa'el (Jihad) Dhiab v. Barack H. Obama et al., Civ. No. 05–1457, US District
Court for the District of Columbia.

18. Timerman, *Prisoner without a Name*, 54.

19. CPT, *Report to the Croatian Government*, CPT/Inf (2014) 9, 24.

20. Carlo Bonini and Massimo Calandri, "La donna kapò di Bolzaneto: Le violenze
e le umiliazioni nella caserma di Bolzaneto" [The woman kapò from Bolzaneto:
Violence and humiliation in the Bolzaneto barracks], *la Repubblica.it*, July 16, 2002,
http://www.repubblica.it/online/politica/gottoventitre/dottoressa/dottoressa.html;
"G8 Bolzaneto July 2001: Italy's Guantanamo Bay," *Indymedia*, March 13, 2008,
https://www.indymedia.org.uk/en/2008/03/393665.html.

21. Amnesty International, *Jordan: "Your Confessions."*

22. CPT, *Report to the United Nations Interim Administration in Kosovo*, CPT/Inf
(2009) 3.

23. CPT, *Report to the Latvian Government on the Visit to Latvia Carried Out by the European Committee for the Prevention of Torture and Inhuman or Degrading Treatment or Punishment (CPT) from 3 to 8 December 2009*, CPT/Inf (2011) 22, July 19, 2011, https://rm.coe.int/0900001680697312; CPT, *Report to the Latvian Government*, CPT/Inf (2013) 20.

24. CPT, *Report to the Government of "the Former Yugoslav Republic of Macedonia" on the Visit to "the Former Yugoslav Republic of Macedonia" Carried Out by the European Committee for the Prevention of Torture and Inhuman or Degrading Treatment or Punishment (CPT) from 6 to 9 December 2016*, CPT/Inf (2017) 30, October 12, 2017, 31, https://rm.coe.int/090000168075d656.

25. Assistance Association for Political Prisoners (Burma), *Darkness We See*, 68, 70.

26. Umiastowski, "Torture in Poland," 41.

27. CPT, *Report to the Portuguese Government*, CPT/Inf (2013) 35, 14.

28. Amnesty International, *Qatar: Briefing to the United Nations Committee Against Torture*, MDE 22/001/2012, October 12, 2012, 3, https://www.amnesty.org/en/documents/MDE22/001/2012/en/.

29. CPT, *Report to the Spanish Government on the Visit to Spain Carried Out by the European Committee for the Prevention of Torture and Inhuman or Degrading Treatment or Punishment (CPT) from 27 September to 10 October 2016*, CPT/Inf (2017) 34, November 16, 2017, 40, 49, https://rm.coe.int/pdf/168076696b.

30. CPT, *Report to the Turkish Government on the Visit to Turkey Carried Out by the European Committee for the Prevention of Torture and Inhuman or Degrading Treatment or Punishment (CPT) from 9 to 21 June 2013*, CPT/Inf (2015) 6, January 15, 2015, 48, https://rm.coe.int/0900001680698344.

31. BMA, *Medicine Betrayed*, 46.

32. Alejandra Dandan, "Los Médicos que Actuaron en la ESMA" [The doctors who acted in the ESMA], *Página 12*, July 23, 2015, https://www.pagina12.com.ar/diario/elpais/1-277713-2015-07-23.html.

33. Solzhenitsyn, *Gulag Archipelago*, 1:208.

34. Steven G. Bradbury, "Re: Application of 18 USC §§2340–2340A to Certain Techniques That May Be Used in the Interrogation of a High Value Al Qaeda Detainee," memorandum for John A Rizzo, May 10, 2005, 16, https://www.therenditionproject.org.uk/pdf/PDF%2016%20[Bradbury%20Memo%20to%20Rizzo%20Certain%20Techniques%2010%20May%20200.pdf.

35. Amnesty International, *Brazil: "They Treat Us like Animals."*

36. Amnesty International, *Out of Control: Torture and Other Ill-Treatment in Mexico*, AMR 41/020/2014, September 2014, 34, 40, https://www.amnestyusa.org/reports/out-of-control-torture-and-other-Ill-Treatment-in-mexico; Amnesty International, *Known Abusers but Victims Ignored: Torture and Ill-Treatment in Mexico*, AMR 41/063/2012, October 2012, 18, http://www.casa-amnesty.de/laender/mex/ai-folterbericht-2012/24106312-CAT-report-mexico-torture.pdf.

37. "Controversy Erupts Again."

38. Albanian Rehabilitation Center for Trauma and Torture (ARCT), *Alternative Report to the List of Issues (CAT/C/ALB/2)*, April 2012, 19, https://www.ecoi.net/en/file/local/1291059/1788_1344869356_arct-albania-cat48.pdf.

39. Devanna, "Maternidad Ilegal de Campo."

40. Voigt and Erler, *Medizin hinter Gittern.*

41. Kingsley and Loveluck, "Egyptian Doctors."

42. Amnesty International, *Syria: Health Crisis: Syrian Government Targets the Wounded and Health Workers*, MDE 24/059/2011, October 25, 2011, 4https://www.amnesty.org/en/documents/MDE24/059/2011/en/.

43. Mikheil Ghoghadze, "Torture Still Happens in Georgia," Democracy and Freedom Watch, April 4, 2012, http://dfwatch.net/torture-still-happens-in-georgia-38857.

44. Koryagin, "Involvement of Soviet Psychiatry," 336–40.

45. Neyyire Yalim and Steven H. Miles, "The Physician and Prison Hunger Strikes: Reflecting on the Experience in Turkey," *Journal of Medical Ethics* 31, no. 3 (April 2005): 169–72, https://doi.org/10.1136/jme.2004.006973.

46. CPT, *Report to the Bulgarian Government on the Visit to Bulgaria Carried Out by the European Committee for the Prevention of Torture and Inhuman or Degrading Treatment or Punishment (CPT) from 25 April to 7 May 1999*, CPT/Inf (2002) 1, January 28, 2002, 15, https://rm.coe.int/090000168069403b.

47. Reis et al., "Physician Participation."

48. UN Committee Against Torture, Concluding Observations on the Fifth Periodic Report of Israel, CAT/C/ISR/CO/5 (June 3, 2016), 4, http://tbinternet.ohchr.org/_layouts/treatybodyexternal/Download.aspx?symbolno=CAT/C/ISR/CO/5& Lang=En; PCATI and PHR–Israel, *Doctoring the Evidence*, 30, 31, 34.

49. Iacopino, *Ending Impunity*, 2.

50. CPT, *Report to the Government of "the Former Yugoslav Republic of Macedonia,"* CPT/Inf (2017) 30, 18.

51. Amnesty International, *Mexico: Surviving Death: Police and Military Torture of Women in Mexico*, AMR 41/4237/2016, June 28, 2016, 40, 41, https://www.amnesty.org/en/documents/amr41/4237/2016/en/.

52. Amnesty International, *Doctors and Torture*; "Nepal: Torture of an 18-Year-Old."

53. Amnesty International, *Peru: Legislation Is Not Enough: Torture Must Be Abolished in Practice*, AMR 46/017/1999, August 31, 1999, 16, https://www.amnesty.org/en/documents/amr46/017/1999/en/.

54. UN Commission on Human Rights, Report of the Special Rapporteur on the Question of Torture, Sir Nigel S. Rodley, Submitted Pursuant to Commission on Human Rights Resolution 1999/32 Addendum Visit by the Special Rapporteur to Romania, E/CN.4/2000/9/Add.3 (November 23, 1999), 7, 10, 12, 13, http://www.refworld.org/docid/3ae6b0970.html.

55. CPT, *Report to the Spanish Government*, CPT/Inf (2017) 34.

56. "Sri Lanka: Another Man Is Severely Assaulted by the Inginiyagala Police," Asian Human Rights Commission, May 17, 2011, http://www.humanrights.asia/news/urgent-appeals/AHRC-UAC-098–2011/; "Sri Lanka: An Innocent Man Was Illegally Arrested, Tortured and Laid with a Fabricated Charge," Asian Human Rights Commission, February 3, 2012, http://www.humanrights.asia/news/urgent-appeals/AHRC-UAC-016–2012/.

57. "Analytical Study about the Leaked Pictures."

58. Amnesty International, *Tajikstan: Shattered Lives; Torture and Other Ill Treatment in Tajikistan*, EUR 60/004/2012, July 12, 2012, 30, 32, https://www.amnesty.org /en/documents/eur60/004/2012/en/; Coalition Against Torture and Impunity, *NGO Report on Tajikistan*, 50–53.

59. Amnesty International, *Thailand: "Make Him Speak by Tomorrow": Torture and Other Ill-Treatment in Thailand*, ASA 39/4747/2016, September 28, 2016, 9, 18, https://www.amnesty.org/en/documents/asa39/4747/2016/en/; Cross Cultural Foundation, Duayjai, and Patani Human Rights Organization, *Torture and Ill Treatment in Thailand's Deep South*.

60. Mary Salinsky, "Torture Continues in Turkey: Findings of New Report," *Lancet* 352, no. 9143 (1998): 1854, https://doi.org/10.1016/s0140–6736(05)79918–9; Amnesty International, *Doctors and Torture*, 1.

61. CPT, *Report to the Ukrainian Government*, CPT/Inf (2012) 30.

62. UN Economic and Social Council, Report of the Special Rapporteur, E/ CN.4/2003/68/Add.2.

63. Amnesty International, *Amnesty International Report 1997—Venezuela*, January 1, 1997, http://www.refworld.org/docid/3ae6a9f818.html; Amnesty International, *Thailand:"Make Him Speak,"* 9, 18.

64. Amnesty International, *Out of Control*, 13, 22, 27, 32, 36, 40; UN Economic and Security Council, Question of the Human Rights of All Persons Subjected to Any Form of Detention or Imprisonment, in Particular: Torture and Other Cruel, Inhuman or Degrading Treatment or Punishment, E/CN.4/1998/38/ Add.2 (January 14, 1998), 22, https://documents-dds-ny.un.org/doc/UNDOC /GEN/G98/101/18/PDF/G9810118.pdf.

65. Amnesty International, *Morocco: Shadow of Impunity; Torture in Morocco and Western Sahara*, MDE 29/001/2015, May 19, 2015, 48, https://www.amnesty.org /en/documents/mde29/001/2015/en/.

66. "Togo: Torture and Bullets Used against Government Opponents," *Irin News*, June 2, 2005, http://www.irinnews.org/Report/54775/TOGO-Torture-and-bullets -used-against-government-opponents-victims.

67. UN Committee Against Torture, Combined Fifth and Sixth Periodic Reports of Argentina, January 13, 2016, 6, http://tbinternet.ohchr.org/_layouts/treaty bodyexternal/Download.aspx?symbolno=CAT/C/ARG/5–6&Lang=en.

68. Colangelo-Bryan and Stork, *Torture Redux*, 147.

69. Assistance Association for Political Prisoners (Burma), *Darkness We See*, 70.

70. Ehab, "Journalists Protest."

71. Jayshree Bajoria, *Bound by Brotherhood: India's Failure to End Killings in Police Custody* (New York: Human Rights Watch, December 19, 2016), https://www .hrw.org/report/2016/12/19/bound-brotherhood/indias-failure-end-killings-police -custody; Bhatia, "Second Autopsy Finds"; Vinod K. Menon, "CBI Books Dharavi Cops for Homicide in Custodial Death," Mid-day.com, January 23, 2016, http://www.mid-day.com/articles/cbi-books-dharavi-cops-for-homicide-in -custodial-death/16889151.

72. Reis et al., "Physician Participation," 1480–86; Lucas and Pross, "Caught between Conscience," 106–14.

73. Assistance Association for Political Prisoners (Burma), *Darkness We See*, 9; "Burma: Police Torture Man."
74. Boo Su-Lyn, "Autopsy Shows 'Torture' but Rules Custodial Death Natural," *Malaymail*, July 9, 2013, https://www.malaymail.com/news/malaysia/2013/07/09 /autopsy-shows-torture-but-rules-custodial-death-natural-surendran-complains /492751.
75. Human Rights Watch, *Peru: Torture*.
76. Umiastowski, "Torture in Poland," 41.
77. UN Economic and Social Council, Question of the Human Rights, E/ CN.4/1995/34, 115.
78. Lizzie Porter and Kareem Chehayeb, "Lebanese Army Accused of Torturing Syrian Refugees," *Middle East Eye*, July 17, 2017, http://www.middleeasteye.net /news/exclusive-syrian-refugees-tortured-death-lebanese-army-481522780.
79. Miles, *Oath Betrayed*, 74–82.
80. Maxwell G. Bloche, *Uruguay's Military Physicians: Cogs in a System of State Terror* (Washington, DC: American Association for the Advancement of Science, 1987); Amnesty International, "Prescription for Change: Health Professionals and the Exposure of Human Rights Violations at 42," app. 2 in *Declaration on the Role of Health Professionals in the Exposure of Torture and Ill-Treatment*, ACT 75/01/96, January 1996, http://hrlibrary.umn.edu/instree/healthprofessional role.html.
81. Amnesty International, *Algeria: Unrestrained Powers*.
82. "India: Detainee Succumbs to Torture by Police," Asian Human Rights Commission, May 22, 2014, http://www.humanrights.asia/news/urgent-appeals/AHRC -UAC-076–2014.
83. UN Economic and Social Council, Question of the Human Rights, E/ CN.4/1995/34, 115.
84. Amnesty International, *Tajikstan: Shattered Lives*, 32; Coalition Against Torture and Impunity, *NGO Report on Tajikistan*.
85. PCATI and PHR–Israel, *Doctoring the Evidence*, 34.
86. Iacopino, *Ending Impunity*, 2.
87. "Mauritania: Torture, Case MRT 030500," World Organization Against Torture, May 3, 2000, http://www.omct.org/urgent-campaigns/urgent-interventions /mauritania/2000/05/d14924/; "Mauritania: Torture, Ill-Treatment and Imprisonment of Haratine People, Case MRT 220800," World Organization Against Torture, August 22, 2000, http://www.omct.org/urgent-campaigns/urgent -interventions/mauritania/2000/08/d14775/.
88. Amnesty International, *Mexico: Surviving Death*, 28, 33, 40.
89. Human Rights Watch, *"No One Is Safe."*
90. CPT, *Report to the Turkish Government*, CPT/Inf (2015) 6, 17.
91. Amnesty International, *Azerbaijan: Torture and Ill-Treatment: Comments on the Forthcoming Review by the United Nations Committee Against Torture*, EUR 55/02/99, 1999, 23, https://www.amnesty.org/download/Documents/148000 /eur550021999en.pdf; Human Rights Center of Azerbaijan and FIDH, *Compliance of the Republic of Azerbaijan with the Convention Against Torture and Other*

*Cruel, Inhuman or Degrading Treatment and Punishment: An Alternative NGO Report to the UN Committee Against Torture*, 2009, 10, http://www2.ohchr.org /english/bodies/cat/docs/ngos/HRCA_FIDH_Azerbaijan43.pdf.

92. Colangelo-Bryan and Stork, *Torture Redux*, 147.

93. PCATI and PHR–Israel, *Doctoring the Evidence*, 32.

94. UN Committee Against Torture, Convention Against Torture and Other Cruel, Inhuman or Degrading Treatment of Punishment: Concluding Observations on the Fifth Periodic Report of Israel, CAT/C/ISR/CO/5 (June 3, 2016), 4, 10, https://www.refworld.org/docid/57a99c6a4.html; "Adoption of List of Issues Prior to Reporting by the Committee Against Torture," PCATI, 2012, http://www .stoptorture.org.il/en/node/1804; Mariam Jishkariani et al., "Session Two: Concurrent Panels: Sessions Involving Marginalized Groups," *Human Rights Brief* 19, no. 4 (2012): 30–31, http://digitalcommons.wcl.american.edu/cgi/viewcontent.cgi ?article=1831&context=hrbrief.

95. Human Rights Watch, *Suspicious Sweeps: The General Intelligence Department and Jordan's Rule of Law Problem*, 2006, https://www.hrw.org/report/2006/09 /18/suspicious-sweeps/general-intelligence-department-and-jordans-rule-law -problem.

96. UN General Assembly, Report of the Special Rapporteur, A/HRC/13/39/Add.3, 43, 48.

97. UN Assistance Mission in Afghanistan and Office of the UN High Commissioner for Human Rights, Treatment of Conflict-Related Detainees: Implementation of Afghanistan's National Plan on the Elimination of Torture, April 2017, 57, https://unama.unmissions.org/sites/default/files/treatment_of _conflict-related_detainees_24_april_2017.pdf.

98. Albanian Human Rights Group (AHRG), Center for Legal Civic Initiatives (CLCI), Children's Human Rights Center of Albania (CIRCA), and Organization Mondiale contre la Torture (OMCT), *State Violence in Albania: An Alternative Report to the United Nations Committee Against Torture*, April 18, 2005, 73, http:// www.crca.al/sites/default/files/publications/First%20Alternative%20Report%20to %20the%20Convention%20Against%20Torture%20-%20Albania%202005.pdf.

99. UK Home Office, *Report of Fact-Finding Mission*.

100. Amnesty International, *Israel and the Occupied Territories*.

101. UN Human Rights Council, Observations on Communications, 105–6.

102. Sarah Dougherty and Scott A. Allen, *Nuremberg Betrayed: Human Experimentation and the CIA Torture Program* (New York: PHR, 2017), https://phr.org /resources/nuremberg-betrayed-human-experimentation-and-the-cia-torture -program/; Miles, *Oath Betrayed*, 186–98.

103. Proctor, *Racial Hygiene*.

# BIBLIOGRAPHIC NOTE

This book must be considered to be a low-resolution picture of torture doctors. A high-resolution picture is not possible. Most information never sees the light of day. The tiny amount that emerges is difficult to find. No nation, human rights organization, or medical association maintains a registry of physicians who have been alleged or confirmed to have collaborated with torture. Few courts or licensing boards make records public, and none have search engines that facilitate searching for torture doctor cases. Journalists haphazardly cover this topic; their postings are often censored, and their websites are annoyingly ephemeral. The brave human rights groups that document medical complicity with torture are often shut down and their websites disappeared. There are no indexes or keywords for searching the general or academic literature. Any piece that contains the words *doctor* or *physician* and *torture* in English or Spanish must be tediously excavated and examined. Most simply describe the account of a physician who has examined a survivor or performed an autopsy.

A few organizations seem especially likely to note physician complicity with torture:

- Amnesty International (http://www.amnesty.org)
- Asian Human Rights Commission (http://www.humanrights.asia)
- European Committee for the Prevention of Torture and Inhuman or Degrading Treatment or Punishment (CPT) (http://www.cpt.coe.int /en/about.htm)
- Human Rights Watch (HRW) (http://www.hrw.org)
- Physicians for Human Rights (https://phr.org)
- UN High Commissioner for Human Rights, Special Rapporteur on Torture and Other Cruel, Inhuman or Degrading Treatment or Punishment (http://www2.ohchr.org/english/issues/torture/rapporteur/)
- World Organization Against Torture (http://www.omct.org)

Two older books focus on physician complicity with torture: Eric Stover and Elena O. Nightingale, eds., *The Breaking of Bodies and Minds: Torture, Psychiatric*

*Abuse, and the Health Professions,* and the British Medical Association, *Medicine Betrayed: The Participation of Doctors in Human Rights Abuses.* Aside from these, there are countless reports, chapters, and articles, as cited throughout this book.

The literature on the human rights movement is far too extensive to list. With sincere apologies to those omitted, at least one of these would serve as the worthy core of any reading program: Lynn Hunt's *Inventing Human Rights,* Juan E. Mendez's *Taking a Stand: The Evolution of Human Rights,* Aryeh Neier's *The International Human Rights Movement,* or Darius Rejali's *Torture and Democracy.*

# INDEX

# ABOUT THE AUTHOR

Steven H. Miles, MD, is professor emeritus of medicine and bioethics at the University of Minnesota Medical School and formerly held the Maas Family Endowed Chair in Bioethics. He previously managed the Doctors Who Torture Accountability Project and is a past president of the American Society of Bioethics and Humanities, from which he received the Distinguished Service Award and Lifetime Achievement Award. Dr. Miles is the author of *Oath Betrayed: America's Torture Doctors*, three other books, and over two hundred articles.

DISCARD